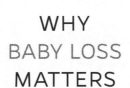

WHY
BABY LOSS
MATTERS

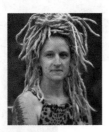

About the author
Kay King is a birth worker and maternity rights activist based in
the South of England. She is the National Coordinator for White
Ribbon Alliance UK, Co-Project Lead for All4Birth and works
to support several leading maternity organisations with strategic
growth, campaigning, fundraising and governance development.
   Kay is also a doula and Grief Recovery Method specialist, who
now focuses on supporting birth within the context of loss. She is
involved in partnership work to deliver and strengthen maternity
education within the context of secondary school relationships and
sex curriculum delivery.

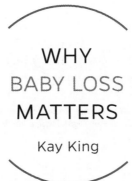

WHY
BABY LOSS
MATTERS

Kay King

Why Baby Loss Matters (Pinter & Martin Why It Matters 20)

First published by Pinter & Martin Ltd 2020

©2020 Kay King

ISBN 978-1-78066-635-8

Also available as an ebook

Pinter & Martin Why It Matters ISSN 2056-8657

Series editor: Susan Last
Index: Helen Bilton
Cover Design: Blok Graphic, London
Cover Illustration: Lucy Davey
Illustration on page 43: Salma Price-Nell at thesalsacreative.com
Author photograph: Mike Pinches

British Library Cataloguing-in-Publication Data
A catalogue record for this book is available from the British Library.

Set in Minion

Printed and bound in the EU by Hussar

This book has been printed on paper that is sourced and harvested from sustainable forests and is FSC accredited.

Pinter & Martin Ltd
6 Effra Parade
London SW2 1PS

pinterandmartin.com

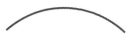

Contents

Author's note

I have made a deliberate choice to include all experiences of baby loss together in one text. I acknowledge that at times this will be challenging, and that your personal experience may align with certain descriptions and not others. Throughout the book I have used the terms 'baby loss', 'pregnancy loss' and 'loss' interchangeably: this is to acknowledge that you can experience loss resulting from the end of a pregnancy or conception journey without feeling that you have experienced baby loss, and that many experience baby loss which has never been validated as such.

I have also used the terms 'women and birthing people', and 'women and families' interchangeably, while acknowledging that baby loss always has the potential to affect all people. Only one experience shared with me for the book was from a transgender person and that person chose to go by the title of woman. At the time of writing there is little specific information available on baby or pregnancy loss directly focused on transgender and non-gender-conforming people.

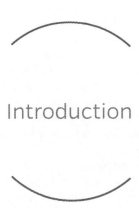

Introduction

Writing this book has brought me into contact with some of the most courageous, brave, honest, and generous people I have ever had the privilege to speak to. Many of them are still grieving and yet all of them were able to find the strength to share their experiences. As I worked to weave together the experiences, words and stories of loss that inform this book, my heart constantly cried out 'No'. Underneath that hearty cry is my recognition that I do not want these words to have to exist: they are sad, uncomfortable, unfair, and hard. I do not want you to have to talk about baby loss any more than any of us want to acknowledge that it is a reality for so many.

But there has and will be power in saying 'Yes' to this opportunity. Power that needs to be returned to the women and birthing people and their families who cannot hide away from the reality of baby loss. Power in the shift in conversation that might begin to occur when more of us dare to look, dare to be in the uncomfortable space that is listening to and caring for people who have experienced baby loss.

As a doula and birth activist I acknowledge that nobody can write the 'right' book on baby loss, for just as there aren't any 'right' words to support people in grief, there aren't the 'right' words to reflect the different experiences that you have faced. The women I have journeyed with and the conversations we have shared have led me to understand some of the simplest things that really do matter, and they are: 'I see you, I am so sorry for your loss and would you like to tell me about your baby?'

Words can be antagonist and balm in equal measure: sometimes carefully chosen words, such as a piece of prose in a ceremony, a poem, or the comforting words of a friend in a letter, can comfort through their delicate placement and intent. Conversely, a badly written email or an insensitive comment on social media can be devastating. Choosing words to soothe grief is subjective, and at the heart of this subject is the unsolvable truth that we cannot quantify or eliminate loss and grief. And yet, while grief is unquantifiable it is also real. For so many people the loss of a baby is part of their life's narrative, never forgotten and rarely soothed. It becomes part of our story in a way that alters everything, in ways far more complex than language has capacity to hold, for it is a matter of the heart, not the intellect.

We tend to talk about baby loss predominantly in relation to the medical definition of what we have faced. We talk about stillbirth, miscarriage, and neonatal death. There can be a tendency to want to understand who we are supposed to blame, or what went wrong. Rarely do we talk about babies, about memories or hopes, or the details of a child, of the difficult decisions we have had to make, of our birth story, the fourth trimester without a baby, our loss of identity, or the impact on the baby's siblings. After the initial event of a baby's death few and precious moments, memories or tactile objects remain to remind us of the existence of a person.

I hope that this book offers you the chance to remember your child, to reconnect to the hopes and expectations that you had for the life ahead of them. I hope that it allows us to unify our experiences of loss in order to better recognise grief and have the tools to hold space for it appropriately. For those of you who have lost something of yourself through the loss of a baby or pregnancy, I hope you feel recognised and less alone.

Baby loss first permeated my work as a doula when I was asked to support a client while she went to hospital for the termination of her pregnancy. I recall her tentative phone call as she asked me if that was '*something you do?*'. At the time I had not considered that as a birth doula I would be with women while they ended their pregnancies, and that a part of my role as a birth companion would be with women through the whole spectrum of conception, pregnancy, birth and loss. Several years and many baby loss clients later I supported a couple as they birthed their stillborn baby at full term. A few weeks after the loss of their daughter my client probed me on why so many books about pregnancy, birth and antenatal preparation omit to mention or expand on the possibility of baby loss. I didn't have an answer. I realised then that loss-holding had somehow been calling me to step more deliberately towards it. As doulas we are not medical professionals; our work is not that of advice-giving, nor is it therapy or counselling. I only know a little about the medical reasons why some pregnancies end, why some babies die and the ways in which these tragic outcomes can be avoided. What I do know is that baby loss matters. It matters hugely and because it is such a complex subject to communicate about and find language for, it has been shunned from many of our conversations about pregnancy, conception, and birth.

This book aims to acknowledge and meet you on a very different journey to the one you probably anticipated when you planned for your children or discovered your pregnancy. It explores grief and healing and offers insight through many first-hand accounts of baby loss. It does not present the 'right' way or the 'wrong' way to manage grief, but rather, as depicted by the beautiful Sufi poet Rumi, my offer is that *'Out beyond ideas of wrongdoing and right doing there is a field. I'll meet you there'*.

According to the Office for National Statistics in 2018 the stillbirth rate in England was 4 per 1,000 births, a decrease from 5.1 stillbirths in 2010. The leading UK-based baby loss charity Tommy's reports that, in the UK, it is estimated that 1 in 4 pregnancies ends in loss during pregnancy or birth. There were 2,958 stillbirths in 2018, and estimates suggest there are 250,000 miscarriages every year in the UK. There were 11,000 emergency admissions for ectopic pregnancies and 2,131 neonatal deaths in 2018. In 2018 there were a total of 200,608 abortions for women resident in England and Wales. These statistics span seven different 'grounds' for termination and it is impossible for anybody to quantify the level of loss experienced by ending a pregnancy.

While statistics offer us an understanding of the scale of the issue, the figures cannot lessen the impact of the loss of a child, and baby loss isn't confined to these given statistics. You might not connect your experience to these statistics and that is fine: in among the numbers it is your loss that matters.

I hope that this book acts to remind us, as birth workers, that loss is part of what we sign up to when we come to this precious and privileged work of holding space for women. When a woman is pregnant, she enters the biggest game of risk, and while we can do everything in our power to ensure that she has choice and dignity in her birth experiences, we must also step up to understand our role in supporting loss.

I also hope that the book acts as a balm to you in your personal loss as a mother or father, a grandmother or father, friend or relative. It is an attempt to offer you comfort at this most difficult time – comfort, but not avoidance. The words and experiences in this book are raw and at times painful to read, but they are presented in a way that intends to bring you closer to knowing that you are not alone. If reading the book is hard at times, step away for a while and come back when you feel ready.

I hope that the book amplifies the incredible work of the organisations and services that strive every day to support the needs of those living with loss. To know where to turn for this support is a fundamental part of healing and grieving, and I hope that this book will be a tool in your pocket, ready to help you or the people you are supporting with baby loss.

As the *Why it Matters* series grows to encompass issues that are vitally important to conversations about birth, parenthood, and the transitional times in between, it is very important that we embed baby loss firmly into the conversation.

To those of you who are choosing to read this book, I applaud your courage. I understand that compassion is an act of courage. May I offer you the compassion you need to turn the next page, to be ready to engage with the conversation of baby loss and for us to work together to change the society we live in so that the language we use to support those experiencing baby loss is part of our colloquial language of love and care for each other.

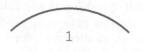

1

Baby loss –
a personal path

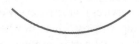

It is dusk and 212 candles sit on my desk, each softly flickering their flame, each representing a life. I have been staring at them for just over an hour, reflecting on the 190 people who shared their loss journey with me. I ceremoniously recall the names of the babies the lights honour, the mothers and fathers they came from and the families they belong to. As I sit in the beauty of their glow, I feel overwhelmed by the unity of these lives, each of them adding to the light of the evening as it closes. It is April 2020 and we are in national lockdown due to the pandemic that shook up the world at the start of this year. Like so many, I am desperate for human contact and desperate to wrap my arms around each of the women and men who have bravely and generously shared their lives and loss with me. I gently whisper the names of your babies: *'Jasper, Luna, Willow, Gracie, Poppy, the Peanut twins, Bodhi, Noah, Indie, April, Matthew...'* I see you; I feel you; you are loved, and you are missed. I recall to my mind every word of every story that has been powerfully shared with me, every loss birth I have supported as a doula and try to capture how I can begin to write a book that is right for you all. I call to mind those of you who will read this book after the experience of a new loss, another loss, or expecting a loss and offer you grace, while willing you great courage as you continue to read. I hold you in the moments of terrifying silence of your grief and I applaud you for your resilience.

Loss and grief are personal journeys, but despite the many theories, psychological understandings and spiritual practices that we have built into our culture in an attempt to understand them, there is no definitive way of doing baby loss 'right'. Grief will manifest differently for us all, and loss and grief change shape in our lives as our experiences and circumstances evolve. There are drastic changes needed to address loss in our society and in maternity care, but I can say with certainty that everyone experiences baby loss in a way that is unique to them. How you come to interpret, acknowledge, define or live with that loss in your life will be very personal. At times it is going to feel, or have felt, as though you are totally alone, that your experience has been forgotten or avoided or shunned by the people around you, and at times it is going to be so present that you might wonder if you will ever be free from its hold. At times you will want never to be free from its hold, because it is the only thing that you have to remind you of the life that was supposed to be there in its place. For others loss will create new meaning in life, perhaps giving you a new path to forge. Baby or pregnancy loss may have left you feeling that you are grieving something of yourself, your identity or past. How you continue to wake up every day and do life without the baby or pregnancy that you carried or hoped for is not predefined: nobody has done it well, or right or better than anybody else, nobody is braver or stronger or worse off than you. Baby loss is unquantifiable and intimate, it is misunderstood and often hidden, it is lonely and can be desperately sad. Every individual experience of it matters.

> *Families, I find, just want you to treat them like any other family you would care for. They want candidness, facts, compassion. Often, they just want to know why; which is sometimes something we can speculate on but often the journey to the answers they so desperately seek is long, and sadly, in many cases of death in utero, none can be found at all. They need to know that there is no 'correct' way to grieve and no 'right' way to respond when they see their baby for the first time, or if they decide not to see their baby at all. It is all valid.* Sophie Simonson, bereavement midwife

Baby loss is experienced in many ways and occurs through a broad range of circumstances. It can be entirely invisible for some, with early pregnancy loss resulting in no physical meeting with your baby, while for others it can occur without your baby having died, but rather having been removed from your care. Sometimes baby loss happens because of planned but not realised attempts at conception, or the breakdown of a relationship resulting in the loss of your parenting role. Some face the heartbreaking decision to end a pregnancy, and some parents face the tragic loss of one of their babies in the case of the loss of a multiple. Your loss experience may be very recent, or it may have happened many years ago. What unifies these experiences is grief and a profound physical and emotional sense of 'missing'. The old English word for grief is 'heartsarnes' and it means 'sore heart'. In many ways it is the perfect way to explain what happens: your heart can feel like it is breaking. Baby loss is a matter of the heart and the heart cannot be healed by intellectual activity alone. You can't read or think your way through grief. Books and therapies and peer support, as well as many other tools, can help you to learn how to live with your sore heart, but the brain is not what needs fixing, and permitting your grief to take its course, led by what you feel, is a new form of learning for many of us. Loss and grief can also cause intense physical reactions, impacting your nervous system, hormones, immune system, sleep and digestion. Understanding your grief and learning how to find peace, connect with memories and identify how you are going to continue a life without your baby may feel impossible, but there are ways, there are tools and I have faith in your strength.

Your experience of grief may be lifelong, or it may fade; it may be peaceful or terrifying. Grief is a response to loss and this will change over time with days and events that feel manageable and others that don't. It will feel hugely unfair and for some it will repeat itself, sometimes more than once. In some experiences somebody or something was to blame for your loss and life afterwards may become consumed by lawsuits and evidence, while for others their loss may be thought by those around them to be their fault. You will feel an entirely unique set of feelings, which may include sadness, depression, terror, loneliness, hope, despair, failure, jealousy and regret. The grief that comes from baby loss is not a linear pathway and there will be emotions that you experience that are interwoven with your personal beliefs, contexts, and previous life events. For some the initial shock of baby loss is overwhelming and all-consuming, while for others the unfolding of the months and years afterwards is when they face their darkest moments.

As a doula I have found that baby loss can carry a silent energy that whispers to others when you meet them, quietly sharing that you have an intimate knowledge of its depth. Perhaps it is this that makes the profound quality of peer support so important in our grief.

When I walked into the room with her, I was so nervous, I didn't want to talk about my loss anymore, it had been four months and I was tired. There were no more words left to say, but when I walked into the room, I looked at her and I knew that she had lost too. Something in her eyes told me that she had also walked this path and that was when I was able to start the therapy work with her that changed everything. She knew loss and right then, that was like a silent hand reaching out and holding my heart. Natalie Delai-Leigh, mother to B

Timescales of loss

When a baby dies, or a pregnancy ends, you may find that your awareness of daily events and activities becomes confused. This is not the case for all women and birthing people, but it is common for families to look back and reflect that time changed, stood still or passed very quickly. It can be extremely challenging to know what to do next. This can extend into not knowing how to continue to care for other children, how to meet your basic needs and how to function in your relationships with others.

The time that you have with your baby, if you get to meet them, will never be enough. It will be brief, and where you expected to have a lifetime of memories what you may actually get can be a blur of heightened emergency, sadness, medical interventions or a short and final holding of your baby in your arms. For many, these precious moments are not possible: perhaps your loss occurred early on, or you had to terminate your pregnancy. Time does not afford you what you and your body were geared up to experience, so what is left is an emptiness, a hole in your story that was supposed to be full of memories and life. You may feel that the pride you have in your baby doesn't receive any audience or acknowledgement.

Baby loss often happens unexpectedly and the medical process can often dominate events surrounding your loss. This is not always the case, and if you have experienced baby loss as a result of many years of attempted conception it certainly won't feel quick or sudden, but for those who expected to be on a nine-month journey towards meeting their child, experiences such as ectopic pregnancy, molar pregnancy and miscarriage can mean that the time between thinking that you were going to be welcoming your baby into the world and facing loss happens very quickly.

When we receive shocking news we are usually given space and time to grieve and recover while we come to terms with what has just happened. The loss of a friend or relative is always very sad, but usually we can take our time to allow that grief to set in, while finding comfort in a life lived. In the case of baby loss, this initial period of grief can be surrounded by a lot of medical decisions and a lot of physical changes in the body of the pregnant woman. It is no surprise, therefore, that you might look back on the time of baby or pregnancy loss and find it difficult to clearly recall the events that took place. You might have a very specific memory, something that somebody said, some physical pain that you felt or a moment that stands out for you. It is important that the people around you understand that you are likely to be in shock, and it is important that you feel able to rely on support from them. If you have a doula or birth partner you might want to ask them to keep track of events. You may wish to go back to your medical records and review events and decisions, find out what caused the loss or seek support by debriefing your birth experience with a bereavement midwife or consultant. As your journey with grief continues you might choose to speak with a counsellor, psychotherapist or grief recovery specialist. You may turn to your faith, seek spiritual guidance, or join peer support groups to meet with others who have had similar experiences.

What our brains take in during times of shock and grief can be surprising and strange. For many, the days immediately after loss hold specific moments and details that stick, while other decisions and interactions are completely forgotten. You might look back on your experience and remember precisely what you were wearing, or the visual details of a particular room that you sat in. You might remember the name of one member of staff at the hospital, or the first thing that your friend or family member said to you. For many there will be an association with a precious object, perhaps your baby's blanket, their crib, a gift or a card that you received. Over time it can feel like these objects are charged with the energy of your grief, holding within them something precious, painful, beautiful or sad. For some women, a specific sensation may remain present for years afterwards: the cold jelly in the sonographer's room, waking up from surgery, or the moment that your baby was placed in your arms.

When we are in shock, our sympathetic nervous system, often referred to as the 'fight-or-flight' mode, is activated and the hormones adrenaline and cortisol are released. In evolutionary terms this sends a signal to our brain to remember the details of the 'threat', so that we can avoid it in the future. It may be, therefore, that the memories that make their way into your long-term memory are the ones that happened when your adrenaline or cortisol levels peaked. Where these subtle but important details remain, you may find that your future triggers are connected to those same sensations. If you experienced trauma during your birth or baby loss you may feel unable to allow your grief to unfold, returning over and over again to the traumatic event and replaying the shocking events in your mind. A recent cohort study published in the *American Journal of Obstetrics and Gynecology* and undertaken at Imperial College in London showed that one month after an early pregnancy loss, of the 737 women studied, 29% had symptoms of post-traumatic stress. This reduced to 18% at nine months. Post-traumatic stress is a reality for a lot of women who experience baby loss and can impact on their ability to begin to process their experience and rebuild their lives. Such stress can also be present for men, family members, birth workers and companions.

As we packed up the nursery and prepared for Liz to come home from the hospital, I found myself going into automatic mode, move this, hide this, stack these away. I was in shock, but this was something to do, she had specifically asked to come home to a clear house. I walked out to the shed to store some of the items and as I opened the door I froze: a highchair that we had been given by a family friend was just inside the door. I had constructed it a few weeks earlier, imagining the day when we would take it out, our baby able to sit solo at our table, strong and ready to eat. I couldn't touch it, couldn't look. I had to ask my mother-in-law to come and move it. I realised then how it must be for Liz, every object that I was stashing away had been pre-loaded with future memories in her imagination, all those things that you think are just practical aids, are actually loaded with hope. Luke, father to Maggie

It is extremely important that the people in supportive, medical, and caring roles at the time of baby loss remain aware and compassionate in their language and sensitivity. So often the memory of one sentence stands out in the minds of bereaved parents, and is it clear these words were insensitive in the context of their loss. Perhaps it is the knowledge of this that makes so many people fearful about what to say. But as with any area of social responsibility and care for others, where we are unsure about what to say, the best course of action is to educate ourselves, equip ourselves with better tools and take responsibility for our fears by learning a new set of behaviours. When supporting people in grief, we will say the wrong things at times, and within reason that is understandable: what matters is that we keep showing up and being there for the person who needs us and that we challenge ourselves to do better. It is likely that you will forgive the odd insensitive comment from somebody who went on to be supportive, compassionate and reliable for months afterwards, and that the people who ended their interaction with you out of fear of saying the wrong thing or in disagreement with your grief will be those that your long-term memory classifies as future threats.

Time can take another strange and painful turn in the months immediately after baby loss. You expected your days to be filled with the continuation of your pregnancy and preparations for birth, or full of the care of your newborn, so the days and nights can become drawn out and empty. The passing of each day becomes both a physical and mental endurance. The irony of the popular phrase 'time is a healer' takes on a new meaning: yes, you may find peace in your life and I am confident that you will, but the time immediately after loss can be overwhelming. It can be extremely hard to know how to fill that time, and for many the first step will be to seek out some peer support from meetings or online forums that can help to connect you with a community of people who will understand your suffering and empathically support you in the early days of your grief. In peer support environments you can see how other people survived the early days after loss. If you have worked with a doula or bereavement midwife you may turn to them for support with your immediate needs. At the back of this book there are resource pages full of services and support groups that you might want to contact.

The value of immediate support

Support after loss comes in many different forms and seeking it can initially feel like a lot of effort. It is completely understandable that you do not want to call somebody up or go to a meeting and face the reality of what has just happened: all you want is for it to be undone and untrue. You may be in shock, having physical symptoms of grief, and be utterly heartbroken, or you may be confused and unclear about how your pregnancy or conception journey has unfolded.

A lack of continuity of care within NHS maternity care, and the medicalisation of birth, means we have moved a long way from the magic connection, empathy, love and concern that is possible between birth workers and women. Unfortunately, the systems, policies and guidelines that inform the way professional health workers operate include professional boundaries which can feel unnatural. We can all understand why these boundaries are there, and yet, while your bereavement midwife may be a great person for you to talk to while in hospital, or in the days afterwards, there is nothing more powerful than ongoing empathic listening and connection from another person's heartfelt connection with your grief, and your relationship with that person needs to feel personal. You may not feel that you have any words, and that you will be in tears or speechless, and this is okay. Many of the support helplines anticipate that people will call them in a state of utter desperation. Other than dialling a number, this step towards support requires nothing from you and can be a powerful first step. One of the greatest things about peer support is a reduced sense of isolation. It allows you the possibility of hearing what you might do with the immediate emptiness, while knowing that there is somebody there who has survived while their heart is breaking.

It is never too soon to receive support. If you need to speak with somebody urgently there are phone numbers, online support groups and charities listed at the end of the book. They are dedicated to listening to you, and their support may be the first step towards lessening your immediate pain.

Becoming a parent

It is common for new parents to talk about when they identified with the role of parent. For some mothers it can be the case that they 'knew' that they were pregnant before they had any hard evidence, and fathers often say that '*She became a mother long before I became a father, that only really happened when the baby arrived*'. It is important to understand that there is no specific moment at which you magically become a parent. Many people feel called to parenthood long before their pregnancy journey begins, while for others that 'natural' parental bond may take years, or even a lifetime, to arrive. Sometimes this can be a fraught issue in couples, with one partner feeling that the other has found parenthood easier or more intuitive. Your identity as a parent when you have experienced baby loss, or the end of a pregnancy, can feel very important. Whether you experienced loss at full term, during neonatal care, or earlier in pregnancy, you may have felt a deep connection to your role and identity as a parent to your child. Only you can define the connection that you felt towards your baby or pregnancy. You may have experienced people taking this identity away from you, or meeting you with the wrong words to describe your experience.

Many people tell me that once they had experienced the loss of their baby, particularly if they did not already have a living child, they felt that people stopped seeing them as parents. That without their baby in their arms, their role as parents was forgotten, lost, invisible, possibly something they would get the chance to be in the future, but not now, without a physical baby to validate that identity. The groups and communities that were once welcoming places of excitement and expectation, such as antenatal groups, pregnancy yoga circles, toddler groups and even groups of friends can suddenly become places of exclusion, with those previously seen as trusted companions suddenly becoming very separate from your daily life experiences. And yet, if an older child dies, we never forget that the parents are grieving their child. The role of parent is never called into question. It is a hard reality to face, when you identify as a parent, that there are people around you who don't refer to your baby by a given name, don't talk to you about the precious details of their short existence, and don't think of you as a parent to your unseen child. If you birthed and met your baby, perhaps were able to feed them, touch them, and bond with them physically for their short, fragile life, you will likely feel a profound sense of pride in your child and birth. Just as with a living baby, asking about how you feel and the circumstances of meeting your baby – who they looked like, what colour hair they had, how much they weighed, whether or not you chose a name – while needing to be navigated with care, can be important to your identity and feelings. After giving birth many women just want to talk to somebody about their baby, and so often the opportunity is denied. To give parents back their identity, despite how they may have been made to feel by others, it is important that we take the time to ask them about their baby as well as their loss. It may be that they do not choose to talk about it – it may be too painful or private – but for those people who are desperate to tell somebody about the baby they expected or gave birth to, not asking denies them their pride and their rightful identity as parents. One client shared with me that a precious experience after her loss was receiving an envelope with both a 'Congratulations on the birth of your girl' card and a 'Sorry for your loss' card. To have a friend acknowledge that two distinct events had taken place and that she had both birthed a baby girl that she was proud of and wanted to celebrate and also experienced the heartbreak of loss, was validating and compassionate.

April, my little girl, was gorgeous. She had a sweet, little face with a cute button nose and pouting little lips. Her fingers were so dainty, and her belly was round and podgy (like mine!). I remember commenting on how long her legs were, despite the ultrasound showing a lagging femur length. She was a little fighter. Her father and I first laid eyes on her on ultrasound during a private 10-week scan. Her little arms waved at us, and her strong heartbeat flickered away, so mesmerising.
Francine Bridge, mother to April

Experiences of loss can occur across the whole spectrum of a conception, pregnancy, and parental journey. While some women birth their babies and are faced with the heartbreak of neonatal loss, others are faced with the devastation of learning of unknown loss in the case of miscarriage prior to knowledge of pregnancy. Many women have experiences that are fraught with the addition of complicated and traumatic decision-making. As I sat with Dawn in the hospital waiting room, preparing for her second termination in two years, we grieved together. *'I just can't stop thinking of this little boy, of how much he wants to come through me into this world,'* she told me. Dawn's circumstances didn't allow for her to have another child. She was already a mother to two older girls, in a complicated court case with one of their fathers, and had such a low income that she simply couldn't afford to have another baby. Her pregnancy was accidental and happened in a very new and unhealthy relationship, but I know that this desperately wanted little boy still visits her regularly in her dreams, plays alongside his older sisters and is loved beyond measure. I know that for Dawn making the decision to end her pregnancy was the right one for her circumstances and her family, but it also came with heartbreak, pain, and careful consideration. To dismiss the loss that she felt, and the grief she responded with, would deny her the compassion that she needed to find peace after reaching her decision and to live her life every day after making it.

Expectation for life

Just as there is no fixed moment or magic switch that defines when we become a parent, there is no exact or fixed point at which a pregnancy, wanted or unwanted, becomes a child in the mind of the parent. It has and probably always will be an area of cultural, societal, political, religious and feminist contention.

Expectations, dreams, hopes and aspirations play a big and special role in the attachment we have to our children and to the role we fulfil as parents. If your pregnancy was planned then it is likely that you engaged in exciting conversations with your friends, partner, or family about the hopes that you had for the new life ahead of you and your baby. If you have children already you had likely considered how the relationship would be between siblings, building an image of your growing family, the fun you would have together, trips you would take, rituals you would share in your home: mealtimes, sleeping arrangements, family cuddles and playing with toys. As a first-time parent you may have already begun to meet with people that would become part of your circle of support, planned groups or activities that you would attend, and spoken with your immediate family about how you planned to parent. An unplanned pregnancy may have meant coming to terms with the life-changing journey ahead of you and building your expectations for your role as a parent. You probably imagined how your baby would look; perhaps you considered what their personality would be like, their features and interests. As we prepare for our expected child, we create invisible maps of how our futures might look, and this magic of the unknown is what can make pregnancy so special. Your pregnancy may also have included physical or emotional symptoms that were difficult for you to endure as your body adapted to carrying the life inside you. If you had the joy of feeling some early movement, you will have begun to bond with your baby's rhythm, your body attuning to their internal touch, their sleeping pattern and active time. You may have spoken to your baby, touched your belly, had strange or altered dreams and maybe even felt that you connected with the soul of the life inside you. In earlier circumstances of loss, you may have been looking forward to these moments, imagining what you would feel, how that would be and what you would enjoy about those incredible moments of carrying a baby. Unless you or somebody close to you has previously experienced the loss of a baby or pregnancy, or you know of potential complications with your own current pregnancy, it is unlikely that in these early days you will have given much thought to the potential for loss. Our minds are, generally, attuned towards hope and the future.

When you experience the loss of your baby or pregnancy

you are thrust into emotional pain that you had very little preparation for. Women facing loss after a previous experience will, at some point in their pregnancy, have been hopeful: fearful too, but hope will have been there and to face another loss is devastating. As humans we seek refuge from our fears and avoid the potential for emotional pain by seeking distractions and thinking positively. If you are fearful of criticism you might avoid putting yourself forward and seek refuge in pleasing others; if you are fearful of failure you might seek refuge by limiting your success in work or relationships. In her book *True Refuge*, clinical psychologist and mindfulness teacher Tara Brach says:

Often it is not until we are jolted by crisis – a betrayal of the heart, the death of a loved one, our own impending death – that we see clearly: Our false refuges don't work. They can't save us from what we most fear, the pain of loss and separation. A crisis has the power to shatter our illusions, to reveal that in this impermanent world, there really is no ground to stand on, nothing we can hold on to. At these times, when our lives seem to be falling apart, the call for help can become fully conscious. This call is the heart's longing for a refuge that is vast enough to embrace our most profound experience of suffering.

Refuge in pregnancy is found in the developing bond between you and your baby. It is this enchanting quality of possibility that allows many of us to remain positive as we endure physical discomfort, sickness, sleeplessness or fatigue. You seek your refuge in the reward: you are to be a parent to a new life. When this refuge is no longer there, you do not automatically switch off your identity as a parent. You are a parent to your baby, and if you feel that your loss, at whatever stage of pregnancy or life, was of your child, nobody should take that identity, that refuge, away from you. Many bereaved parents are not given this with the power and recognition that it deserves.

Finding a path towards compassion and empathy for baby loss which challenges our own beliefs requires us to recognise that the point at which somebody considers themselves to be a parent is personal and unique. Of course if you are legally the parent of a living child there are different considerations and arrangements, responsibilities and requirements that you must navigate; whether or not you have 'felt' like a parent takes on a different context when there is a living child to be nurtured. In the case of baby loss, however, it is not for the observer to judge whether the expectation for life creates in us an identity as a parent. That sense, feeling, perception or identity as a parent to an expected life, conceived or not, is personal and should not be questioned, but rather validated. People experience the relationship with their unborn baby, sometimes their unconceived baby, in completely different ways. I have known women who have experienced multiple miscarriages who do not think of those losses as their children, and I have known women who have grieved an early termination for years, missing their baby and with deep conviction identifying as a mother to that child.

I was 32, and in a very intense relationship with Jason. We were living together in Manchester, along with his six-year-old daughter. Six months into our relationship her mother died in an accident. Three months later I was pregnant. My first known pregnancy. Totally unplanned, and in the emotional aftermath of a huge loss. My period was late and by the third week, with breasts so sore I couldn't bear to be touched and overwhelming fatigue, taking a test was only confirming what I already knew. I couldn't stop smiling when I saw the double lines on the test: my body works! I love children and can easily engage most of them, I never had the urge to have my own but finding myself with one growing in my womb threw up all kind of emotions. My partner didn't want the baby. I was mother to his bereaved daughter, yet he rejected the child we made together. I felt rejected as a woman. He'd had three previous terminations with girlfriends and was accustomed to abortion. I didn't want to have a baby with a man who didn't want it. Penny Penman, mother to Matthew

It is so important that we recognise that the more we can ensure every parent has their feelings of loss validated, the more companionship and compassion we can offer them in their grief and the more likely they are to feel supported and recognised. Nobody chooses to experience grief, so when it is present in your life being equipped with the tools of validity and recognition, consideration and kindness will allow you the best chance to survive and find peace. Baby loss is unfair. Sometimes baby loss happens multiple times in a person's journey and that is hugely unfair and extremely sad. To lose a child at any stage of pregnancy or conception goes against the natural order of life, in which parents are supposed to die before their children. The loss of a baby can feel deeply unnatural and as though your body and mind are unprepared to handle it.

Try not to lose all connection with the hopes and dreams you had for your life with your baby. When the time feels right you could write these down or record them to listen to in the future. These are your memories for a future unrealised: they are what charges your love and what makes your heartbreak so real. While remembering them and going through the act of putting them into words may feel raw and painful, one day those same words may act as physical reminders of your baby.

Empathy and sympathy

A common thread between all circumstances of baby loss is that people have to navigate difficult relationships with those around them while they are grieving. Hannah lost her baby due to an ectopic pregnancy when she was 36. Her relationship with her mother had previously been very close; they lived near each other and her mum would have been involved in both the birth and the day-to-day childcare. Hannah says:

Mum refused to let me grieve. She wanted me to heal, to be okay, to get over it and try again. I was devastated and couldn't understand why she couldn't see that and let me take my time to heal. The constant message was that it was unlucky, that I would get pregnant again and that this baby probably just wasn't meant to be. Mum scorned my idea of having a funeral for my baby and it eventually led to a breakdown in our relationship. We were at a wedding a few months later and when I referred to the loss of my baby while chatting to a family friend, Mum got really embarrassed and butted in with 'it was ectopic so not really a baby'. I remember being completely wounded by her perspective on her grandchild.

Empathy towards another person's feeling around loss can be really challenging. You may be very close to that person – perhaps you are their partner, their mother, their friend or their ex-partner – and have very different feelings about the same events. You may have both experienced a miscarriage and one of you is feeling that there was no loss, while the other is distraught and grieving. Or perhaps you have made a joint decision to end a pregnancy and one partner feels that this is a liberating decision that improves their life, while the other is sad and maybe experiencing some regret. The important leap that we need to take in order that every person in every circumstance is validated is to step beyond our own feelings and acknowledge that while we may not understand it, their emotional response has value. This is not easy: emotional empathy is such a complicated concept that many people dedicate their life's work to it. Marshall Rosenburg, the late American psychologist, developed a world-renowned process called non-violent communication (NVC) that aims to achieve emotional empathy through communication with others. In NVC people are invited to communicate through a four-stage process in which they observe the event that has occurred, identify their feeling about that event, attach that feeling to a need and then make a request for how the other person might help them meet that need. It is a complex, yet revolutionarily simple technique, and it underpins my personal understanding of how important empathy is when we come up against challenging emotions. In practicing NVC in my own relationships and in my work as a doula and parent, I have found empathic listening to be one of the greatest challenges. To really listen to somebody, and to silence the quiet judgements, opinions, and beliefs that you hold, takes work and practice, but it is deeply rewarding and a transformational tool for anybody who finds themselves supporting somebody through loss.

The ability to take the perspective of another person, particularly if you yourself are directly impacted by that perspective, is the biggest challenge of empathy. Empathy is all about connection, about standing with another person and seeing exactly what might be going on for them, feeling into their pain because of your care and concern for them. Learning to act out of empathy for others takes courage, humility, and grace. Sympathy has its place, and in the circumstance of baby loss it is often what people lean towards, but when it is offered as a substitute for empathy it can also fuel disconnection. Sympathy is about acknowledging a person's misfortune and feeling sorry for them and for their situation; it sits closely alongside pity and when it comes to baby loss, pity can be toxic.

When you meet somebody who has experienced baby loss, being well equipped with empathy is important. You might not agree that they have experienced baby loss: you might think that they chose to terminate their pregnancy, or be confused because they were never actually pregnant. You might have experienced the loss of your own pregnancy or baby and feel that your experience was very different from theirs. It can be really challenging to shift away from our own judgement and support a person who has had a different experience to ours. Grief does not have the same rules for everybody and where some people take very scientific approaches towards understanding life and death, others may experience these same concepts spiritually or through a personal faith. Some people find themselves to be extremely pragmatic in circumstances of loss, while others remain deeply affected by the aspirations and hopes that they had for their child. Empathy enables you to put aside your own perspective and really hear what is happening for the other person, and then meet their need for support.

Saria had wanted to have children for five years. She felt called to be a mother, and that she and her partner were in a place in their lives where having a baby was right for them. They had been married for nine years and she was in her late thirties when, after four rounds of IVF treatment, they made the decision to stop trying. Saria had been unwell with each round and needed to focus on her own health. She told me:

I have four babies that didn't make it. They each have a name, they each have an intended birth year, they have a bedroom in our home, I am their mother and yet nobody will ever see me as a parent.

Imagining the life ahead of our babies, for many mothers and families, is as much a part of the transition into parenthood as conceiving them, caring for them and raising them. When these expectations do not result in the physicality of parenthood, the identity that has been formed must be given the dignity and respect that we would give to any parent.

If you have experienced grief as a result of baby loss, at whatever stage in your pregnancy journey, and you are grieving your baby, then it is important that you feel allowed to grieve for the child that you carried, held, hoped for or expected.

Eventually they disconnected all the wires and I could finally hold him in my arms. He lived for about 20 minutes. His breaths slowly getting more infrequent. The odd shudder as his body started to shut down. And eventually I realised he was gone.

After he died, I stayed with him for most of the day. We took prints and casts of his hand and feet. I was able to give him a bath and dress him. In fact putting him in his babygro I picked him up to my shoulder and said 'there we go, that's better' and suddenly I was overcome with sadness and cried properly for the first time that day.
Lois Darcy, mother to Bodhi

The grief that you feel

> *Grief is not a negotiation with death, it is a glorious love letter to life.* Azul Valerie Thomé

Maybe it is because we live in a culture that promotes positive thinking as a signifier of mental wellbeing, or maybe it is because it is instilled in us as children to appreciate what we have, not what we don't, that grief has suffered from our cultural tendency to look beyond our circumstance and find a 'worse' one to compare it to. Many parents who are experiencing baby loss share their feelings of not having it as bad as others. It is common for parents to say *'I know it's not as bad as their experience, but…'*. We have so much information about other people's experiences these days that the tendency of the human mind to compare ourselves to others is increasing. Living with loss in a digital world opens us up to comparisons of grief: in every forum we join, every support group we engage in, we become one among many. While this can have many benefits, there is also a risk that we lessen our personal experience of loss when we hear many other stories and allow ourselves to constantly compare our grief to others. This can be especially true if you seek peer support exclusively online and in the form of an observer, rather than as a participant. While online support can be incredible, to receive support there is a requirement to participate, to ask, to share and to engage. This can feel really hard and exposing, and it is a big step to speak and share your grief, although it is also one of the bravest and most significant steps towards working with your grief. A combination of face-to-face peer support and online support can help you to receive support as well as observe it.

The Grief Recovery Method presents an interesting insight into grief comparison that I have found to be very useful in the context of baby loss: all grief is experienced at 100 percent, there are no exceptions. The grief that you feel is *your* 100 percent. Your grief is your experience and it cannot be diminished by comparing it to others. There are many factors that underpin this theory, one of which is that the way that you experience loss is directly linked to the degree to which you felt emotionally complete with that person before they died. Feeling emotionally complete in relation to the life you expected your child to have is what we seek when we try to get pregnant. For the pregnant person, our hormones and bodies begin to shift and change to form an attachment and bond in preparation for our role as carer to that child. Emotionally incomplete describes how we can feel when we say goodbye to a baby, whether that pregnancy was planned or not. Feeling a sense of emotional incompleteness when we experience loss, of a pregnancy or baby, or a part of our physical body in the case of ectopic pregnancies or hysterectomies, is entirely understandable. How our grief manifests for us on a personal level is our 100 percent experience of it. It is never helpful to be met with people who try, despite their best intentions, to move you away from your grief without acknowledging it. Grief is a response, not a singular emotion, and the idea that we would disallow, limit, or dismiss somebody's response to loss, takes away their autonomy. Supporting you to recover should come after acknowledging that you are grieving. Attempting to quantify, compare, fix, or dismiss anybody's grief does nothing towards their recovery or healing.

Family and friends said the same things as before, only this time there was the added 'third time lucky' and 'it'll happen when the time is right' but for us, the time was right. We wanted that baby. And the first one too. Instead we just had loss and empty places in our hearts. Elizabeth Martin

To permit yourself your own grief is also important, and it is likely that you will not know what this will look like from one day to the next. With so much comparison to others it is very possible to diminish your own grief by telling yourself that you are not as entitled to it as another. I have met many mothers who experienced baby loss years ago who have said that it was not the 'done thing' to grieve for their baby. This silencing, possibly a very British 'stiff upper lip' hiding of our experiences, has done very little to heal women who have been encouraged to quash their experiences of baby loss, keep quiet and carry on. Your grief might not seem as 'big' or 'tragic' as somebody else's, and it may not have come alongside trauma, but if it is there, I encourage you to seek support to talk about your experience, if for no other reason than to seek a deeper sense of peace in your life going forward.

For some people, the end of a pregnancy does not resonate with the definition of baby loss, and for those people it is also okay to acknowledge that their experience was very different. An early miscarriage for one person may be an event of very little significance, something that 'had' to happen in order for their living babies to come into being, or something that gave them the opportunity to realise that having children wasn't right for them. You may have reflected on a previous loss and recognised that the timing wasn't right for you or that child, and define your experience very differently to others. You can experience the loss of a pregnancy and not identify with having experienced baby loss, and you can experience baby loss without ever having been pregnant. One experience is not comparable with another: even when the medical or gestational experiences are the same, the associated emotions, responses and definitions are entirely personal paths. What we must move towards supporting is the grief, seeing the person and their feelings rather than the sequence of events.

I was made to feel that because I didn't meet my baby, because I didn't birth a baby, my loss wasn't as bad. I still hurt. My feelings are still valid. I still had to pass things and 'birth' things. I had to push my pseudo sac out. It wasn't much of a push. But I still had the bearing down feeling. I still needed to push. That was emotionally painful too and my feelings are valid. Loss is loss and pain is personal. You are still allowed to grieve your baby if you lost it earlier than someone who had a still birth at 40 weeks. Yes, they'll be hurting... It doesn't mean you can't hurt. It doesn't mean you can't and shouldn't grieve. Kelly

You may have experienced baby loss and other pregnancy losses and be aware of how they differ in terms of your emotional perception and response. This is perfectly normal. None of the experiences are your fault, nor are they fair and how you come to define and signify one loss should not be comparable to any others. Just as no two relationships between parent and child are the same, no two circumstances of loss will bring the same journey of grief. Words and care and healing choices that applied to your situation in one loss may be totally inappropriate for another.

What is grief?

In 1969 psychiatrist Elizabeth Kubler-Ross wrote a book entitled *On Death and Dying*. This presents grief through a framework of five stages and was written in relation to grief after being diagnosed with a terminal illness. The stages of grief she identified – denial, anger, bargaining, depression and acceptance – were presented as an emotional pathway. The popularity of the book led many people to apply this staged response to grief in all circumstances. Ross went on to publish another book with David Kessler called *On Grief and Grieving*, in 2005. It adapted the five stages of grief model to accommodate new perspectives on the non-linear nature of grief. However, the original 'five stages' became commonly accepted, despite the fact that in the event of loss, you are unlikely to follow any fixed pathway. While it may be felt by some, it is very unlikely for example that you will experience 'denial': baby loss is very real, and I am yet to meet a bereaved parent in denial about their loss. You have probably heard people refer to a friend or relative as 'going through the stages of grief', and if you have experienced baby loss you may have come across people who comment on which stage of grief you are currently in. The five-stage model was ground-breaking at the time, but more recently other stages have been added by scholars, psychologists and therapists, including shock, guilt, and pain. There is now a wide range of progressive and individualised approaches to grief.

Thus there are problems with many of the colloquial words that we associate with grief, such as 'process', 'stages', 'going through' and even the word 'recovering' – we now see that staged emotional pathways or processes, whereby you start at one end in shock or denial and gradually arrive at acceptance or recovery, do not take into consideration the deep and personal complexity that exists for each individual. So while the original five-stage model is still often referred to, please don't accept anybody telling you what 'stage' of grief you are in. Your emotions are your own, and while it can be enormously helpful to work with a professional to identify, name and work through them, you are not simply following a defined model of behaviour or response. Your grief will be yours, unique, hard, and interrelated to all your other life experiences.

Imagine trying to control somebody's response to anything else in life: your projections and interventions could be considered coercive, controlling and limiting, and would potentially act to silence the other person. Of course, there are many examples of where this happens in life and society: we shame, embarrass, control, quash, cover up and dismiss people's responses to many things, but outside of necessary protection of confidentiality, or the safety of ourselves or another, it is never right to be corrective about how somebody responds to something that has happened to them.

Mum said to me, 'you haven't reached anger yet'. She was so sure that I was at the point when that was meant to kick in – like I was a textbook case. My baby died, I wasn't angry, because I am not an angry person. I ain't never been angry, and now it's four and a half years later and I'm still not angry. Don't think I am not sad, I can't tell you how sad I am. Jamie was meant to be celebrating his fifth birthday this year, that is really sad. But Mum was wrong, I am certainly not sitting around waiting for the anger to kick in! Laura, mother to Jamie

Owing to the unique and personal way in which grief impacts our lives, there are some words that you will resonate with and some that you will not. There are also some words that are commonly applied to grief which are worth exploring because they have a habitual, unconscious tendency to seep into our language and they carry with them some real problems. The word 'closure' is one: it suggests that at some point you will find a way to close part of your story down. You may have heard people say 'At least now they have closure' at the end of a legal investigation into baby loss, but I guarantee that the people they are talking about do not have any such thing. They may have a medical answer to why their baby died, but they will be no more complete emotionally. They may have answers, clarity and in some cases justice – but they do not have their baby. Two other words that are often used are 'victim' and 'survivor'. Throughout this book I refer, at times, to your need to survive and this is deliberate to highlight that for some people, grief can make you feel that you do not want to live anymore. In those darkest moments, with all my compassion, I want you to survive and find the resources you need to feel able to live. But there is no point at which you become a 'survivor' of loss: you are somebody to whom this experience has happened and you are living with, recovering from or finding peace with your grief. Another challenging identity is that of 'victim'. No, you are no victim. You have not been harmed or injured as a result of a crime or an accident, and being given the identity of 'victim' does nothing to acknowledge the incredible amount of emotional hardship you may face, nor the incredible strength that you have. And you are incredible: you may not feel it, but living with baby loss, putting one foot in front of the other, going on with your parenting of other children, potentially facing and overcoming the fear of future pregnancies… that is not 'victim', that is powerful, resilient and strong.

'Recovery' is another complicated word and there is a shift required in our thinking to realise that there is a big difference between forgetting and recovery. When you experience baby loss you will never forget your baby. When you experience any form of grief you will not forget that you have had those feelings or challenges in your life. However, loss of a life lived affords us the grace of the memories of a person's imprint upon the world, while baby loss leaves a quieter, less visible imprint on your heart. My work in grief support has led me to wholeheartedly believe in the possibility of recovery and the hope for it after baby and pregnancy loss. The problematic relationship with the idea of this resides not in the potential for recovery, but on what we have, through our education and associations with the word, come to believe that it is.

Recovery does not mean that you will never be sad, or that you are 'over' your loss. It does not mean that you will not have pain or days that feel terrifyingly dark. Recovery means that you can feel better, that you can come to share your experience of loss and grief and consider this healthy and normal. Recovery is being able to talk about your sadness without being affected by the impact of it on other people. These things are possible: I have seen them happen for many women and families.

There is hope for recovery through finding ways to connect with the love that you feel for your baby and being joyful about the short, sweet memories that you have of them. In many ways I think we all believe in recovery – it is why we seek support, and why we strive for healing. The key to recovery, I believe, comes from understanding how we can begin to feel emotionally complete again, and this requires the right techniques, emotional work and caring support.

The circle of grief or 'ring theory of Kvetching'

When a baby dies or a pregnancy or conception journey ends, or indeed whenever we are facing challenging, sad or traumatic experiences in life, knowing that the people who are closest to you will provide you with the support you need is essential. There is a lot of fear present with the subject of grief and people can find it extremely difficult to know what to say, how to say it and how to avoid offence. If you have experienced baby loss you are likely to have had at least one, if not many more, experiences of people insensitively bringing their experience of your loss to the forefront of their interactions with you. These exchanges may have been intended to be delivered as acts of support or sympathy for your situation, but sometimes phrases such as *'I just cannot believe that this has happened'* or *'I don't know if I can handle this'* can bring increased grief and sadness to your experience, adding the weight of other people's emotions to your load.

Susan Silk is a clinical psychologist from the United States who, through her own experience of breast cancer, developed a simple technique called 'ring theory of Kvetching'. This technique is also sometimes referred to as the 'circle of grief' or 'circle of support'. Kvetching is a Yiddish word that means 'to habitually complain'. It refers to complaining or grumbling about something repetitively or habitually. This is not what grieving people do when they are sharing their experience with others, so you could replace the word with 'share' or 'offload' or simply 'grieve' to better apply the definition to this context.

Ring theory works like this. You draw a ring and in the centre you write the name of the person who has experienced the loss first-hand. In the case of baby loss this is the person who is or was pregnant, or who was trying to conceive. You then place another ring around that person and in it you put the person who is closest to the person at the centre, perhaps their partner. You then add another ring and continue to put in the people who are closest, perhaps siblings, grandparents or close friends. You continue this process of drawing rings and positioning people depending on their relationship to the person at the centre of the circle. The person at the centre of the circle is allowed to say whatever they want to whoever they want in the wider circles. They have the right to 'Kvetch' and complain as much as they need to – that is the one pay-off for being at the centre of the ring. Everybody else can also complain and 'Kvetch', but only to people who are in rings *outside* their own. Whenever you talk to somebody or share with somebody in a ring *inside* your own, you do so to help them, not to receive help for yourself.

This simple theory can have a demonstrable and supportive effect for all involved. It prioritises the person at the centre of the trauma, while ensuring that everybody can share and receive support for their pain and grief. If you are currently supporting somebody who has experienced baby loss, or indeed any form of loss or trauma, it may be useful to pin an image of the ring of grief in a place that you regularly look. By reminding ourselves that we need to 'dump out' our emotions to the wider rings and bring 'comfort in' towards the centre, we can move towards a support cycle that ensures nobody is responsible for the emotional weight of other people as they try to navigate their own response to loss.

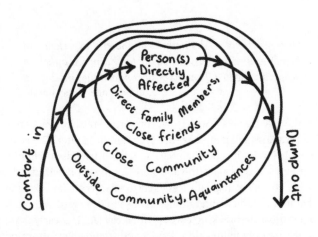

How to draw a ring theory diagram

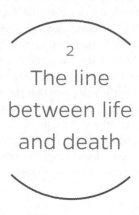

2

The line between life and death

Our reluctance to honestly examine the experience of (aging and) dying has increased the harm we inflict on people and denied them the basic comforts they most need.
Atul Gawande, *Being Mortal*

In the UK there is a widely accepted rule in early pregnancy that we don't tell people we are pregnant until after 12 weeks, at which point it is deemed 'safe' to tell our friends and family our news. It is a rule with valid statistics to support it: after 12 weeks you are statistically less likely to miscarry. It is also a rule that many women and families choose to disregard, although often this rule-breaking comes with a caveat: 'It is early days, so we are only telling close family and friends'. Let's examine what we have set ourselves up for. While it may still feel right for you to keep your pregnancy private for the first trimester, it is worth considering that in doing so we also set ourselves up to face potential loss in increased isolation, unable to source the support that we might need. Sometimes we adopt societal 'norms' just because they are 'normal' and 'what everybody else does'. We don't always consciously examine why we have chosen to follow suit. The first trimester of pregnancy tends to be the one with the most physical symptoms, so keeping your pregnancy a secret during these months may be an additional challenge.

The question to ask yourself when deciding whether you are going to share your pregnancy news is: who are you protecting, and from what? If you were to experience baby loss, who would you need for support? If you would feel comfortable sharing a potential loss with friends and family, then it is also fine to share news of your pregnancy. Without sharing your news, will the people around you be able to build their own expectations and hopes for that life? And without these, will they be able to share in any genuinely empathic grief with you if you experience loss? It can be very challenging to grieve empathically for something you never had knowledge of.

One in four pregnancies in the UK ends in a miscarriage. That figure astounds me, regardless of how often I hear it. It doesn't feel like that many, because they pass us by in secret. The invisibility of baby loss in our society is partially linked to the fact that we are actively encouraged to keep our loss a secret from others. It is surprising, when discussing pregnancy and birth with very close friends, to discover that they experienced a miscarriage which they did not tell anybody about. While I'm not advocating for all miscarriages to be publicly announced, we do need to feel able to share our stories of loss if we need support to recover. Imagine a world in which we could say that we had experienced a miscarriage and others were able to meet us with empathy and compassion, rather than being speechless and feeling awkward. That shift will only occur as we begin to challenge what is 'normal' in our pregnancy journey. Perhaps sharing happy news, with the risk of it leading to a loss, is something that we could collectively be more responsible for. If you want to tell people you are pregnant, and are also prepared to tell them about a loss, then it is completely up to you to share your news whenever it feels right.

No word for you

In the book *My Sister's Keeper*, author Jodi Picoult writes *'In the English language there are orphans and widows, but there is no word for the parents who lose a child.'*

Identity is something that we all seek. Titles, qualifications, job roles and names are all ways in which we state to others 'This is me, this is my context'. And yet in the English dictionary there is no word for a bereaved parent. This might not be important to you; you may wish to be referred to as the parent of your baby and be happy to share with people who meet you about your loss. But for others, the lack of a word to describe your experience of baby or child loss leads to a life of explanation that can be tricky and clumsy, leaving you to explain repeatedly the details of your experience. If we meet somebody and they tell us that they are widowed, we can meet them with sensitivity and compassion – we understand that they have experienced loss. If given further detail – 'I am recently widowed' – we know that it is likely that this person is still deep in their experience of grief. We have a colloquial context for that person without having to ask them more than they are willing to share. Imagine if a recently widowed person had to explain every time: 'My husband/wife died recently and I am still grieving and therefore sensitive to loss and conversations about death'. It would be a painful disclaimer at every new introduction. The common understanding and acceptance of a singular word protects the individual from having to explain. But for a parent who has experienced baby loss, no such word is widely accepted. There is, however, a Sanskrit word that has been adopted by many westerners. Sanskrit is an ancient Indo-Aryan or Indic language, in which there are many words that the English language does not offer. In the case of baby loss, the word 'vilomah', which translates as 'against a natural order' has been used to describe a parent whose child has died. A few years ago, a bereaved parent started a petition to get the word into the English dictionary because she felt so passionately about its use for her experience of grief. Whether or not you feel you need a word, it is worth noting that one of the reasons why we may struggle to receive the care and support that we need when we experience baby loss is because we don't have words to describe it. A client and friend whose baby was stillborn, when talking to me during her pregnancy with her second baby, said:

So me and Dad have both been added to this Mum's and Dad's group, called 'Becoming Parents', and it has made us both feel really confused and a bit angry that we are seen as 'becoming' parents, when we already are parents to our daughter.

It is so often in the subtle exclusions of society that we find ourselves most reminded of how invisible our grief is when it comes to baby loss.

A death-denied society

In 1984 Professor Allan Kellehear, a sociologist who writes about death and dying, wrote a paper presenting the idea that we are a 'death-denied' society. Further study into the 'taboo' of death, and how society in the UK has informed our engagement with death, has been done by Tony Walter, a researcher in death studies at Bath University. I do not mention these to suggest that when you experience baby or pregnancy loss you should become fascinated by the academic study of death in society, but my experience of working alongside families tells me that you will come to experience a broad sense of denial from those around you. The dominant reaction to grief and death is fear and awkwardness. Rarely does it seem that we have accepted death as commonplace and a subject we feel comfortable sharing. In his work Tony Walter states that 'death is nature threatening culture', and I see this in the experiences of my clients when they share their sad news with those around them. People are threatened by death, their experience of culture is threatened, and they do not have the tools, exposure, or direct experience to know how to meet their friends, partners, or colleagues in their grief.

The hardest part about returning to work was facing Jenny, my pregnant friend and colleague, who sat in the next seat. From time to time someone would come over to talk to her about her glowing complexion or how often the baby was kicking, and if I wasn't feeling strong I would just get up and walk to the photocopier, or go and make a cup of tea. I tried my best to deal with scan photos being passed around, and pregnancy announcements from other colleagues, but it was hard. The trauma of the birth was still pretty fresh in my mind, even eight weeks on, and my heart broke a little more each day as my friends grew more distant. One day, my closest work friends took me to a café to tell me it was too hard to support both me and our pregnant friend, so from then on they would just be there for her, and if they said anything inconsiderate then they were sorry, but they were tired of filtering themselves. Christina Clarke, mother to Poppy+4

We live in a society that like things that are clean, things that promote happiness and success and things that can sell. We also live in a society that has in many ways been led by and for men. Baby loss isn't exactly a shiny concept: you don't see pictures of it, don't find stores lined with products that can support it and we don't live in a culture that makes a point of highlighting that it happens. Women have experienced generations of silencing of their baby loss. Perhaps it is worth considering that baby loss has been overlooked by much of society because it is predominantly a feminist issue. Of course grief affects men, and yes we are fortunate to be living in an age of increased equality, but in a historically patriarchal society the experience of pregnancy and pregnancy loss has been sidelined as a 'women's issue'.

Grief can be dark and confusing, and it can be present for a very long time. It informs how we live going forward and changes our way of seeing and being entirely. That much of society chooses to ignore it, feels threatened by it and shunts conversations about it into counselling rooms and support groups is symptomatic of how much emphasis society places on progress, moving on, economics, capitalism and growth. Western society has a strained relationship with death and dying: we don't like to dwell on things that make us feel uncomfortable, which require us to learn and change our ways, and we don't like to give up or lack hope, or admit fear or failure. This is true of all areas of medicine and end-of-life care, not just baby loss: we are a society that likes to fix and heal, cure and solve. We advance wellbeing at all costs and strive to eliminate death from disease; we spend ever-increasing sums on research to preserve and prolong life. The message to us all is that death should be avoided as much as possible. It is understandable that we don't want people to die, but it is also inevitable. The unfortunate result is that we put very little resource, thought and research into how we hold and support a society that does and always will experience loss.

Baby loss carries its own unique challenge in a 'death-denying' society, which is that it does not often come with an association, for those around us, to a physical person. It may be possible to grieve alongside somebody who lost a relative that you shared. You may be able to go and visit their grave together, place flowers and hold annual ceremonies for the date of their birth or passing. When life ends at an old age, we can understand the natural order of it – although it is sad, it makes more sense and we hold on to the celebration and memory of a life lived. This is not the case with baby loss. Often there is no grave, no funeral, and very few memories that can be shared. There is little physical evidence of our baby in our lives, beyond knowledge of a pregnancy or attempts at conception. In some cases of baby loss we aren't even talking about an issue of physical death: many women lose their babies in other ways. Their baby is alive but has been removed from them or separated from them in some way. To know where to put the grief in these tragic circumstances goes against what our bodies and hearts can comprehend.

I believe all situations where a mother loses her baby are crucially important – above all else, times when compassionate, sensitive and individualised maternity care should be a priority. Each situation will be different, each mother will want and need specific approaches to her care and midwives and maternity workers should first of all listen. Listen to her, her family and try to comprehend the circumstances surrounding the event. Midwives are in a prime position to support mothers and families with sensitivity and tact, avoiding language that may trigger guilt or shame – or deepen the emotion. If a mother has her baby forcibly removed, try to remember she is still a mother. Imagine her unspeakable grief when her body is still responding physiologically and psychologically to the birth and her baby being with another carer, out of her sight. I can still recall the screams of one mother as her breastfed baby was plucked from her arms. It continues to distress me. Kindness and love are the best tools for support, and we can be the ones to share it. Sheena Byrom OBE, midwife

Signing up to life and death

The morning after I arrived home from the hospital having supported a couple through the birth of their stillborn daughter who was born at 28 weeks, I sat in my garden on the phone to my doula mentor Maddie McMahon, and author of *Why Mothering Matters*, and reflected on the experience. I had supported loss before, but none that had happened quite so suddenly, and I was in shock. The labour had taken 18 hours and we spent several hours afterwards holding their daughter, looking at her fingers and toes, her delicate features, giving her a name and all of our love. I remember Maddie's words so clearly:

We forget that this is what we sign up to with this precious work, that it is always a line between life and death. Whilst so much of our work is based on the joy, the choice and dignity of birth and parenthood, what we also sign up to is a gamble of life and death.

She was right, I had forgotten. My client's pregnancy had been a joy to support. I was so excited for them to meet their daughter and so delighted by her empowered approach to her birth that I had lost sight of the potential of that gamble. Holding her baby was a privilege that I will never forget, and it was also a time during which I felt my role as a doula most powerfully. I didn't have to *do* anything, but I had to *be* there, enduring with all my courage my role of being with woman. In all of the pain and sadness it was completely about the couple and their daughter, and putting aside my fear so I could be present with them in their grief powerfully tested my understanding of being a birth doula.

When we sign up to supporting women and birthing people as doulas, midwives, doctors, health professionals and birth keepers, we are entering into a fragile form of magic. For all the medical progress that we have made to ensure that we minimise the chances of baby loss wherever possible, it still happens, and it always will. To fully engage with the responsibility of what our work calls us to as birth workers we must educate ourselves on the experiences that women and birthing people may face. Our responsibility to continue to learn, and to lean into that learning with an open mind and brave heart, is vital to developing empathy.

Supporting a person through any life transition is a huge honour and responsibility. I am therefore keenly aware that when I welcome a group of prospective doulas into their learning space I am duty bound to make sure that not only do they feel safe to talk about loss, but are adequately prepared for the possibility that they may encounter families whose babies die during their work as doulas.

Whether a trainee doula has endured the loss of a baby herself or not, most new doulas come into this work with fears around loss. They may be scared of being triggered if their clients miscarry or have a stillbirth, or they may fear not knowing what to say or do if a client is bereaved. The first step is always to maintain a safe, supportive space so that new doulas can express these worries and fears. If they have lost a baby themselves, they may benefit from doing some deeper trauma work in preparation for supporting their clients. For others it is enough to talk through some scenarios, speak with doulas who have supported families through the loss of a baby and gather their resources and signposts so they have a rich and supportive toolkit to offer the families they serve.

The most important thing is to teach doulas to always remember the orbits of support. At the centre is the person going through the trauma of loss. Everyone around that person sends love and support into the centre, but must remember to look outwards for any support they may need for themselves. This means the doula should spend time and energy building their support network so that they have strong arms to hold them should they need support. Maddie McMahon, founder of Developing Doulas

All birth workers are duty-bound to recognise that we sign up to the potential of supporting people with baby loss. If you have experienced a loss in your own conception or pregnancy journey and are working to support women and birthing people within your work, I encourage you to address your own grief first. That does not mean that you need to be healed, or beyond your grief, to support others – indeed, a deep empathy exists between women and bereavement midwives and doulas who have themselves experienced loss. But before you start educating yourself on how to support others, please ensure that you have created your own circle of support.

Although I hope that you don't face loss in your work, many of you will, and to be prepared to continue in your role with the compassion that is needed, you need to have worked with your own grief as a priority.

National Bereavement Care Pathway

One of the first steps in this learning might be to undertake a course or read some books about baby loss. Another essential aspect of our work should be to familiarise ourselves with the National Bereavement Care Pathway (NBCP) for pregnancy and baby loss. Launched in 2017 and led by the charity SANDS, backed by the All Party Parliamentary Group on Baby Loss, the NBCP sets out standards that are now being adopted by trusts across the country and are also being delivered in Scotland. The pathway is based on a set of nine bereavement care standards which can and should be adopted by all NHS trusts. The bereavement care standards are:

1. *A parent-led bereavement **care plan** is in place for all families, providing continuity between settings and into any subsequent pregnancies.*
2. *Bereavement care **training** is offered to staff who come into contact with bereaved parents, and staff are supported to access this training.*
3. *All bereaved parents are informed about and, if requested, referred for **emotional support** and for specialist mental health support when needed.*
4. *There is a **bereavement lead** in every healthcare setting where a pregnancy or baby loss may occur.*
5. ***Bereavement rooms** are available and accessible in all hospitals.*
6. *The preferences of all bereaved families are sought, and all bereaved parents are **offered informed choices** about*

decisions relating to their care and the care of their babies.

7. *All bereaved parents are offered opportunities to **make memories**.*

8. *A **system is in place to clearly signal** to all healthcare professionals and staff that a parent has experienced a bereavement to enable continuity of care.*

9. *Healthcare staff are provided with, and can access, **support and resources** to deliver high quality bereavement care.*

NBCP Pathway website

The NBCP had its second review in 2019, when 32 trusts across England had piloted the pathway. While the overall evaluation highlights positive improvements in bereavement care within NHS maternity settings, there is still a long way to go for these standards to be available across all trusts. One of the areas for improvement highlighted was:

High-quality bereavement care for parents who have ended their pregnancy after a prenatal diagnosis or had an early pregnancy loss is still often a challenge as care is provided away from a maternity setting. Trust leaders need to pay attention to the quality of all bereavement care, and how the NBCP can support the delivery of effective care in these settings. Fiveways Evaluation of the NBCP, May 2019

It is important to recognise that while the efforts being made through the NBCP deserve praise, the journey of grief extends outside the maternity care setting. Having signposts to services that can support women and grieving people in the months and years after their experience of baby loss is also important, and we can all work to build connections with the incredible services and charities striving for this ongoing care.

If you experience baby loss in your role as a birth worker, you can ask to speak with the bereavement lead in a hospital setting and ensure that you utilise the support and resources on offer in your trust. In a sector which is about mutual support for all families and birthing people you could get involved in supporting your local trust to ensure that the standards are being rolled out in your trust. Working with your Maternity Voices Partnership or signing up to volunteer for a loss service or charity will help to ensure that progress is being made within bereavement care.

If you have experienced baby loss yourself or have recently found out that your pregnancy will result in loss, these standards should be your expectation for care within your NHS trust. If they are not available within the setting where you are due to give birth or have already given birth you can ask your midwife for support from a trust that is offering these standards of care, or you can contact one of the loss charities in the resources section of this book to ask about where you can go to expect these standards of care for you and your family.

Training and techniques for supporting loss

There are several ways that birth workers can add to their professional development and increase their ability to best support loss. These tools and techniques are also beneficial if you are experiencing your own grief after loss. No therapeutic technique or course will be right for everybody and you might, as you begin to navigate your grief, find that you don't like a particular approach, and that is okay. You never have to endure something that doesn't feel right, although pretty much every experience of support around loss will involve feeling uncomfortable and painful at times. As you seek the right support for you, ask yourself whether you are just feeling inevitable pain, or whether you want to try another technique because this one is not helpful for your individual circumstances. Having an honest and open-minded perspective will help you avoid skipping from one technique to the next seeking answers. None of these approaches will bring your baby back, none of them take your loss away, and often they require perseverance to really reap the benefits.

3-Step Rewind

The 3-Step Rewind is a technique used to neutralise disturbing feelings associated with trauma. While not exclusively designed to deal with loss, and not a technique that deals with the long-term nature of grief, it can be extremely valuable for women and birthing people for whom loss included trauma. You may have experienced baby loss after the shocking discovery of finding your baby when they died, or you may have experienced a very traumatic surgery or birth. With the 3-Step Rewind the memory of the event will still exist, but the associated anxiety, panic, guilt, sadness and anger can be eliminated. There are three stages:

- Deep relaxation
- Recalling the event in a specific way while feeling safe and secure
- Imagining coping in the future and responding differently

In my experience, the 3-Step Rewind can help immensely with the traumatic feelings associated with baby loss, rather than a method for managing grief. While grief is an ongoing response, feelings that we may describe as traumatic are usually associated with moments, or events. It can be hard for a parent to tell their story, when it's so full of trigger points that cause distress. This can leave them 'stuck', so they find it difficult to move forward. The practitioner guides the client into a deep state of relaxation, where they are able to reprocess the memories, and lift some of those difficult feelings. It is not a treatment, rather an activation of their ability to self-heal. The process can be carried out months or years after a bereavement with similar results. The parents I have worked with often report 'relief' after the process, when these traumatic feelings are lifted, and the distress reduced. Many midwives (both independent and NHS) and doulas are now trained in the 3-step Rewind, with many offering the service remotely, so finding a practitioner is easy. Ellie Cook, Birth and Postnatal Doula NLP Master Practitioner, 3-Step Rewind trainer

Consider 3-Step Rewind if you are troubled by feelings associated with a specific memory or event from your experience of loss. Trauma and grief are two quite different things and sometimes acknowledging that the trauma is the block to moving forward is key to unlocking your pathway towards healing.

I went straight to hospital and was told that I'd got constipation and to rest and go home, as it was common to feel those symptoms after a miscarriage. Two days passed and I started to haemorrhage and was blue-lighted to hospital. My body was still registering a pregnancy but after overnight observations I was allowed back home. What followed was the most traumatic experience. Within a couple of weeks, I haemorrhaged again and was sent back to hospital. I endured another anaesthetic and having that fear that I would die on the operating table consumed every part of me. The day after I was told that I had retained placenta, and this is what my body was rejecting, all the remains of the previous pregnancies. I was informed that I was so badly infected that the doctor was surprised I was here at all. It was then that I took up my concerns with the hospital and was personally visited by the Head of Midwifery. She stated that the D&C [dilation and curettage] *that was carried out was a non-viable pregnancy and that all I had lost was just some cells. I remember saying 'But I've got a scan picture,' to which she said 'Go and get it for me, I want to see'! To have to sit there and prove that I was pregnant and that my baby was of the gestation, it was truly terrible.* Joanne Sieber

The Grief Recovery Method

The Grief Recovery Method was created over 30 years ago by John W. James and is a useful tool to explore how we work with grief resulting from any form of loss. It uses the following definition and explanation of grief:

Grief is defined as the 'conflicting emotions that follow the ending or change in familiar patterns of behaviour.' This complex emotional state has nothing to do with our intellect. We cannot rationalise ourselves better. Therefore any 'treatment' that appeals to our heads and not our hearts is doomed to fail.

The Grief Recovery Method is:

- not counselling
- not therapy
- not an alternative treatment

It is a process which brings new understanding to the word 'recovery' and seeks to find ways to regain a sense of peace in your life, while never forgetting what or who you have lost. The Grief Recovery Method can be undertaken by following the *Grief Recovery Handbook* (details in the resources section at the end of the book), or you can contact a Grief Recovery Specialist and work alongside them, undertaking activities and techniques that will help you find your own path to recovery.

Closing the Bones

The Closing the Bones ceremony is commonly used to support new mothers after the birth of a live baby. It is also incredibly powerful for women who have given birth or been pregnant and experienced loss. Many doulas and birth workers are trained in how to provide the ritual.

> *Closing the Bones is a way to support a woman's recovery after childbirth; a way to celebrate the amazing abilities of her body; and a way to create a moment of stillness, of meditative peace and reflection in the rollercoaster of emotions. It is a postnatal ritual. It is a ceremony. It is a massage with warming, nurturing use of a shawl or scarf. However she birthed her child, this is a time to breathe, reflect on her journey so far and feel loved and supported by her community.* www.closingthebonesmassage.com

While many postnatal experiences become unavailable for women facing baby loss, and there is exclusion from feeling able to attend group postnatal classes, meetings or social gatherings, the Closing the Bones ritual can be hugely welcoming for a mother or woman grieving. They will have experienced the same or similar physical changes to their bodies as any woman with a live baby, so a space where their commonality rather than glaring difference can be celebrated and nurtured can be extremely valuable.

You can train to deliver the ritual if you are a health worker, doula, birth worker or body worker. If you have experienced pregnancy or baby loss and feel that you would like to be supported with a Closing the Bones ceremony and massage there are many practitioners who can offer the ritual in your home or a private space.

Supporting Every Birth

Doula and mentor Michelle Every offers a course called Supporting Every Birth for doulas and birth workers, which provides an opportunity to consider caring for yourself as a birth worker, valuing every birth, including loss, and learning from those who have experienced or supported loss. This course is now exclusively offered through Nurturing Birth doula courses and is a valuable addition to any previous or future doula training.

Spirituality and faith

This world can seem marvellously convincing until death collapses the illusion and evicts us from our hiding place.
Sogyal Rinpoche, The Tibetan Book of Living and Dying

It is easy to overlook our impermanence as humans. Modern life is concerned with the acquisition of more, of better, of upgraded material possessions. The message is very convincing and it is easy to buy into the illusion that death is a far-off concept as we strive for better jobs, bigger houses, and more and more physical objects. This becomes very clear when you experience baby loss: suddenly the impermanence and fragility of life is brought to our attention in the most vivid and painful way. Death and grief can take over very suddenly and our hearts and minds are unlikely to be prepared for their darkness. Sometimes the contemplation of life and death has already had significance in your life: you may have experienced the loss of friends, relatives or a partner, or you may work in a sector that brings an awareness of human fragility into your day-to-day consideration. If you have grown up with a faith or philosophy that informs your opinions and thoughts on death and life you may find that these beliefs are extremely valuable and comforting during your experience of baby loss. For others, these very beliefs are called into question and you may find yourself challenging some of your previous convictions now that you are experiencing the loss of your own child. After the loss of a baby or pregnancy, or as you grieve the end of attempted conception, you may find that you seek solace and comfort in a new faith or philosophy. Baby loss brings us into contemplation of the non-physical presence of another being in new and extraordinary ways. It is likely that you will spend a lot of your time after your loss remembering the expected or short life and character of your baby.

The word 'spiritual' gets bad press. One definition of the word is that it is relates to religion or religious belief, and for many of us this excludes us from identifying with being 'spiritual'. However, there is another very inclusive definition which is relevant to us all: 'relating to or affecting the human spirit or soul as opposed to material or physical things'. Using this definition, baby loss is a spiritual happening. To relate to that which is not physical is a spiritual experience and you may find that after the loss of your baby, pregnancy or conception journey, your mind is regularly attuned to that which is no longer physical.

To come to spiritual contemplation because of baby loss may present you with feelings that you have never spent time exploring. You may have gone through life without witnessing loss before and find yourself contemplating non-physical existence for the first time. You may already contemplate spiritual realms, and find that baby loss brings you back to some of your previous thoughts. For many bereaved parents there is comfort in the knowledge that their baby has a soul, a spirit, or an energy that remains present in their lives and that they can spend time connecting with. However you choose to do this, whether through meditation, ceremony, prayer, ritual or just spending time recalling your baby, there can be huge benefit to keeping a spiritual connection with your child.

I expect some people would regard me as naive or trying to protect myself when I say that I felt the Peanuts [name given to the twins] *wanted to die in my womb. But I do know myself well and know my own truth. The Peanuts were due on my husband's birthday, and the day they were due we conceived my youngest daughter. She was due on the birthday of my deceased best friend. When I had the termination, I had a vision of my children on the beach with me in India, I had the same vision when in labour with my youngest. The birth was very powerful and very different from my first, after seeing the Peanuts in the vision I landed bang into my body just as my youngest daughter passed through me into this world. That feeling of landing in my body gave me a sense of power grounding and confidence that I'm still carrying, and I've never had before. For me all these things are significant and powerful, and they all connect me with my babies. The Peanuts are buried in our garden and when my youngest daughter was born, we buried her placenta there, to watch over them. For me it is important that they were given back to the earth. There is a bench next to them and I talk to them often when really happy or sad and if we go away, I like to go and check in with them when we come home.* Alice Caudle, mother to the 'Peanut Twins'

Sometimes the idea of spirituality can be better understood through considering energy exchange and the physics of our human energy. In June 2005, physicist, writer and journalist Aaron Freeman, on National Public Radio's *All Things Considered* show, read the following, which has come to be known as a 'Eulogy from a Physicist'. This is an extract from the full piece and speaks profoundly to the continuation of energy after loss.

You want a physicist to speak at your funeral. You want the physicist to talk to your grieving family about the conservation of energy, so they will understand that your energy has not died. You want the physicist to remind your sobbing mother about the first law of thermodynamics; that no energy gets created in the universe, and none is destroyed. You want your mother to know that all your energy, every vibration, every BTU of heat, every wave of every particle that was her beloved child remains with her in this world. You want the physicist to tell your weeping father that amid energies of the cosmos, you gave as good as you got.

And the physicist will remind the congregation of how much of all our energy is given off as heat. There may be a few fanning themselves with their programs as he says it. And he will tell them that the warmth that flowed through you in life is still here, still part of all that we are, even as we who mourn continue the heat of our own lives.

And you'll want the physicist to explain to those who loved you that they need not have faith; indeed, they should not have faith. Let them know that they can measure, that scientists have measured precisely the conservation of energy and found it accurate, verifiable and consistent across space and time. You can hope your family will examine the evidence and satisfy themselves that the science is sound and that they'll be comforted to know your energy's still around. According to the law of the conservation of energy, not a bit of you is gone; you're just less orderly. Amen.

Whether or not you come to a particular faith, philosophy, science or belief about where your baby has 'gone' when you experience baby loss, there will likely be times when you find yourself connecting with the potential that their existence, or hoped-for existence, brought to your life. Your baby's spirit, soul or energy can continue for you in whatever way you deem most appropriate, and ultimately in the way that allows you the most peace.

Yet grief is common to all humans and what fills me with a second grief is that our society does not acknowledge this. We don't have the words. I believe grief however painful brings important lessons connecting us with something bigger than ourselves. An understanding that we are not in control. Grief and love are two sides of the same coin, when I feel grief in my body it feels like love ... an aching full heart. My grief would not exist without love and my grief teaches me to embrace love in the knowledge that it will one day move into grief. Alice Caudle, mother to the 'Peanut Twins'

Avoidable circumstances of loss

Any circumstance of baby loss is extremely sad and will feel hugely unfair in your personal life. Many of the leading baby loss charities in the UK strive to ensure that research is being undertaken to find new ways to reduce instances of baby loss. This work is vitally important for families for whom future or further loss can be avoided.

There are some statistics that relate to baby loss, however, which are not dependent on medical advancements or the need for greater understanding of the physiology of pregnancy, but rather that relate to the inequalities and vulnerabilities created by society. Some of these statistics stem from systemic inequalities in healthcare provision and some from relationship environments. Birth activists across the UK strive for a reduction in humanly avoidable instances of baby and maternal loss and there are certain issues which require urgent change.

Inequalities for minority groups in maternity care and baby loss

The National Maternity Review, *Better Births*, (2016) sets out a five-year plan for recommended improvements in NHS maternity care. The review states:

> *Our vision for maternity services across England is for them to become safer, more personalised, kinder, professional and more family friendly; where every woman has access to information to enable her to make decisions about her care; and where she and her baby can access support that is centred around their individual needs and circumstances.*

The *British Journal of Midwifery* reported in May 2020 that:

Black and black British women have an increased risk of stillbirth in the UK. The stillbirth rate for the UK in 2017 has reduced to 3.74 per 1,000 total births. However, mortality rates remain high for Black or black British women, despite stillbirth rates for these groups reducing over the period 2015–2017 from 8.17–7.46 per 1,000 births. Draper et al, 2019

The reasons for this unacceptable inequality in health outcomes are multifactorial and a thorough review of the care available for Black and black British women is desperately needed. We can also see that UK stillbirth rates are in part dependent on human action, rather than genetic or medical advancements. The Department for Health identified one of the reasons for inequality: '*An inability to access antenatal care is known to lead to increased infant mortality in black and minority ethnic women.*' (Department of Health, 2010).

I went in on a Monday morning and I could feel it all around the room, I felt like I was causing a massive fuss. It was early in my pregnancy, around 14 weeks, and here I am causing a fuss about something that everybody would rather not be dealing with. The voices and tone of the nurses made me realise that they thought I was a bit of a nuisance! I don't think they liked my boyfriend either, nobody made any eye contact with him or said they were sorry for either of us. I've never been with anybody else when they lost their baby but if this is how everybody is made to feel it is all wrong. The doctor said to me 'It is not unusual, don't be too upset' and then walked out the room. It felt like I had been slapped across the face. And you know, of course I am going to question if this was the way I was treated, because I am me, my skin is brown,

67

and I am made to feel like I am overreacting. It's just there, always, it's always there, either that or the whole system is broken for women who don't get their babies.
Kari Nahra, mother to L

Tragically, the inequalities in maternity care for Black, black British and minority ethnic women do not only impact stillbirth rates. A report from MBRRACE (Mothers and Babies: Reducing Risk through Audit and Confidential Enquiry) highlighted that in the UK, from 2014–2016, black women were five times and Asian women twice as likely as white women to die in pregnancy and childbirth. It is evident that disproportionate adverse maternity outcomes are seen in BAME (black and minority ethnic) groups. Currently, maternity services in England are predominantly a one-size-fits all, and many marginalised women have difficulty having their specific maternity needs met.

Baby loss is unforgettable and unfair, but baby loss resulting from increased risk due to unaddressed systemic racism within maternity care is unforgivable. No one should feel more at risk of baby loss due to disproportionate standards of care. Where inequalities exist, they should be addressed as a matter of urgency. If you experienced loss due to substandard maternity care your grief will be amplified by the injustice. My work as a birth activist has afforded me the great privilege of working alongside many organisations, charities and people who are working tirelessly to bring about change, and while there is a long road ahead to secure commitments that will result in better outcomes, please know that you are not alone in your suffering and that many wonderful, devoted activists and birth-keepers are standing up to the injustices, systems and people that have caused you heartbreak.

The injustice of baby loss for black women, and steps we can take to improve maternity services

It is incumbent on maternity services to reduce stillbirths, but also to provide safe care and support where stillbirth has very sadly occurred.

Given prenatal attachment, the death of a baby in the womb is a significant event for any woman, and her partner and family. In supporting them, we recognise the critical physical, emotional and psychological aspects of their care. Needs will vary in intensity, volume and stages, from the first knowledge of baby's demise, right through until when support is no longer needed.

Given the intransigent and long-standing burden of stillbirth in the community for people of African descent, much thought needs to be given as to how to best give support that meets their needs and values. The significant disparity in outcomes between this community and their white counterparts – stillbirth rates are around 50% higher – is a serious cause for concern.

It is true that the issues are complex and point to systemic and multiple causes. Many calls are therefore made for more research to examine and explain the causes, with a view to making recommendations. However, in my continued years of patient and public involvement, I have noted some dissonance in approach to the problem. 'Hard to reach' is the term used by service providers, while the communities mention their frustration at having to 'make do' with the services available to them.

Utilising the concept of 'intersectionality' gives us insight into the lives of childbearing women of African descent. We are able to see how stillbirth, both at the personal and

the strategic levels, profoundly and unjustly impacts these women, their partners and communities in many far-reaching ways.

Putting the woman at the centre of her care, so she is able to choose safe services, recognises that people of African descent are not a homogeneous group. Solutions begin with 'listening' to women, 'hearing' them, respecting and meeting their needs and values. The 'continuity of carer' midwifery model has proven itself over time as making an immediate and profound difference to stillbirth statistics.

In the sad cases where stillbirth occurs, we then need effective professional, relevant support from culturally safe services which have been developed and commissioned with a 'bottom-up' approach. Without a bold and courageous approach to action these principles we miss another opportunity for reproductive justice in our maternity services.

Elsie Gayle, practising midwife, community researcher and strategic advisor to maternity services.

Domestic abuse and baby loss

In 2018, domestic violence prevention charity Refuge reported that 20 percent of their service users who were victims of domestic abuse were also pregnant. Between four and nine women in every 100 are abused during their pregnancy or shortly after they give birth. Tommy's is the largest charity funding research into the causes of miscarriage, stillbirth and premature birth. It highlights that during pregnancy domestic abuse increases the risk of miscarriage, premature birth, low birth weight, infection, physical injury to the baby and even death. Many people, including victims, think that domestic abuse is only violence, so reading the official government definition may be useful:

Any incident or pattern of incidents of controlling, coercive or threatening behaviour, violence or abuse between those aged 16 or over who are or have been intimate partners or family members regardless of gender or sexuality. This can encompass, but is not limited to, the following types of abuse:

- *psychological*
- *physical*
- *sexual*
- *financial*
- *emotional*

Controlling behaviour is: a range of acts designed to make a person subordinate and/or dependent by isolating them from sources of support, exploiting their resources and capacities for personal gain, depriving them of the means needed for independence, resistance and escape and regulating their everyday behaviour. Coercive behaviour is: an act or a pattern of acts of assault, threats, humiliation and intimidation or other abuse that is used to harm, punish, or frighten their victim.

Information for Local Areas on the change to the
Definition of Domestic Violence and Abuse www.gov.uk

You should be asked about your relationship circumstances at least once during your maternity care. It is a requirement that every pregnant person is given the opportunity to disclose, in a safe and private environment, exposure to or experience of domestic abuse. Many people who are experiencing abuse may not want or be ready to leave the abusive relationship, and no assumption should be made that by disclosing to professionals, agencies or friends, that you will be pressurised to leave. What is important for any victim or suspected victim of domestic abuse to know is that you can get support that is focused on your needs and circumstances.

Domestic abuse is very common (according to the Crime Survey for England and Wales for the year ending March 2019, an estimated 5.7 percent of adults (2.4 million) experienced domestic abuse in the last year). Domestic abuse often starts in pregnancy and poses risks to the unborn child, and statistically there is a link between domestic abuse and infant mortality. Those working with pregnant women have a duty of care to routinely ask about abuse. Victims need to know that they are not alone, will not be judged and that there is help available. Statistically women experience up to 35 incidents of abuse before they seek help, and contact up to 11 agencies before they receive the support they need.

Pregnant women who have separated from their abusive partner need to agree a birth plan with their midwife, doula, or other birth attendant and state clearly who they want present at the birth and who they do not. Abusive ex-partners often turn up at maternity units and manage to wheedle their way in. A detailed birth plan ensures all professionals know who should and should not be present.

Maureen Wells is an IDVA (Independent Domestic Violence Advisor) who works with high risk victims of abuse in Northamptonshire. She offers the following insight into the context of baby loss and domestic abuse:

If someone is experiencing domestic abuse and has suffered a miscarriage or stillbirth or neonatal death, their abuser is unlikely to allow them to grieve and may even use the situation as an abusive tool i.e. you're not fit to be a mother, you killed your baby. They may not allow them to speak of their child's death or, conversely, keep mentioning it or talking about it, not allowing the victim to move on.

There can be the added fear for the pregnant woman that disclosing an abusive relationship or environment risks their baby being removed from their care. The fear of unwanted intervention from social services is very real for many women and can mean that they remain in an abusive relationship despite knowing that it is not a safe environment for them or their child. For some women the relationship may feel inescapable due to financial or coercive control that makes them fear for their lives. If you have experienced baby loss resulting from domestic abuse your grief will be amplified by your circumstances and you may continue to experience abuse during the fourth trimester, or indeed for years after the loss of your baby. Please know that there are services available to help and protect you. There are several resources at the end of this book that will help you or ask a friend or family member to contact a service that can support you.

In my work I have walked the pathway of loss, I've witnessed the threat of loss, and sat with the aftermath of loss of a child(ren) with women who have suffered systematic abuse by an intimate partner. The harmed partner finally reaches a place where they can leave the abuse, however in the UK if a father/partner's name is on the birth certificate they are automatically gifted something called equal parental responsibility (until a family court can decide if this right should be removed). This essentially means that a perpetrator of intimate partner violence (without police convictions) who has their name on a child's birth certificate can exercise their equal parental rights and could withhold a child or children from you and the law protects them to do so. There are many tragic and devastating stories of courts awarding full custody to a perpetrator of harm. We sadly have a long way to go for the first response services to understand the often complex situations that exist and for our family court service to operate in a way that prevents continued abuse of one parent at the hands of another. Katie Olliffe, Independent Domestic Violence Support and doula

Leaving abusive relationships can be tremendously difficult and the loss of your baby or pregnancy as a direct result of domestic abuse is tragic. Nikki, who lost her baby through heartbreaking experiences of domestic abuse and coercive control, shared the pain of her loss with me as she described some of the abusive behaviour she experienced:

He was the most beautiful little boy and I was so excited to take him home and enjoy feeding him and dressing him in all the beautiful clothes we had been given and watch him sleep in the lovely Moses basket all sweetly decorated. I had and have never experienced such elation in all my life. Those feelings will never die in me. I was so in love with my new baby. I loved to bathe him, breastfeed him and rock him to sleep in fluffy towels. It was such a joyous time. These precious moments were to sadly be cut short. Me and my new baby were not allowed to bond. The controlling behaviour crept in from Yasim. He began to tell me how to do things and that I didn't know what I was doing. He would tell me that my son never smiles with me and only him and showed me some pictures and made me feel like this was so. He began to control me more and more about the housework and again I would retaliate at the injustice. Until one day he came into the bathroom with a large knife and threatened to kill me. I ran downstairs through a door into the downstairs shop.

I stood at the back of the shop shaking in a towel asking for the police to be called. The police came and took me and my baby to the police station.

Nikki's life with her son came to a very sad end a while later, and many years on she has found the words to share her experience and the impact that losing her baby has had on her life.

I have spent my life hurt by all of this and have struggled to fit into a 'normal world' despite my efforts. The love for my child helped me get off heroin, go to university, get a career and be 100 percent committed to him despite our strangeness. He was sadly poisoned against me and struggled to respect me. We are now close after many years and my son is sad that I went through this. He has an allegiance to his father and that can never be broken. My baby remembers the knife when I first tried to leave with him and so he believes me, which is far more important than all those grown-ups who didn't. I tried to reclaim my Motherhood by having a child through IVF at 42 but it failed. I am now grieving this, but it doesn't compare to the pain of grieving the child I had stolen from me through domestic violence and not being heard as a victim.

Baby loss resulting from abuse is avoidable and requires that we, as a society, continue to strive for excellence in our care provision, that we practice and support with due diligence in the vital safeguarding measures required for our role and have awareness of the services and charities that exist to support victims at any stage of their journey.

Change and action

Your experience of baby or pregnancy loss, resulting from inequalities in your maternity care or vulnerabilities in your relationship, may lead you to feel motivated to join in with the action driving change in these areas. You may feel so deeply in your personal grief that activism, campaigning or hearing more about others suffering is just too much and it is certainly not your responsibility. Either way you should address your personal need for care, support, healing and strengthening your own health as a priority. Your grief should be nurtured, and you need to be held through your pain without having to expose yourself to even more of it.

However, some women and families feel called to social action after the loss of their baby and have enormous drive to get involved in work to help reduce future suffering for others. If this is you, there is information about some of the projects and campaigns in the resources section.

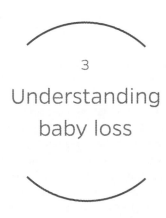

3

Understanding
baby loss

Many of the leading baby loss charities focus on raising awareness. In 2002 the first Baby Loss Awareness Day was organised by a group of bereaved parents. Since then, with support and backing from many UK charities, the day has grown into a Baby Loss Awareness Week that takes place annually in October. Raising the awareness of baby loss means that we want more people to know that it happens, that there are things that can be done to reduce how often it happens, and that more support needs to be made available for women and birthing people and their families. This collaborative effort amplifies the fact that baby loss is still overlooked, misunderstood and in many cases invisible.

You may have come to understand baby loss as a result of your own experience, or that of somebody close to you, or you may be about to face a pregnancy after loss or be reading about loss because of your work as a birth worker. Part of my work over the last few years has been in Relationships and Sex Education for young people. In September 2020, in England, the National Curriculum on Relationships and Sex Education became a mandatory part of what schools must teach our children. With a curriculum that focuses heavily on preventing teenage pregnancy, avoiding sexually transmitted diseases and upholding family values, even this new strand of our children's education makes maternity care and baby loss relatively invisible. In some school biology textbooks there are references to ways in which a pregnancy can end, and within our contraceptive education, from a family planning clinic or in school, we may learn about termination of pregnancy, but there are so many ways in which a woman or birthing person can experience baby loss that without any formal or informal education it is no wonder that the subject remains largely unseen. Abortion and teenage pregnancy continue to be viewed as shameful by society, and many young people begin adult life feeling silently guilty, shamed or a failure, without ever being supported in their grief for a life lost.

With that in mind, although I attempt to highlight many of the ways in which you may have come to experience baby loss, this chapter will not capture them all. The most important thing to remember is that your grief, your experience of loss, has value. You have interpreted the loss of your pregnancy, your unmet expectation or hope for conception or your separation from a living baby as baby loss, and you are allowed to grieve and be comforted. You should be treated with respect and kindness by those around you.

Miscarriage, stillbirth and neonatal loss are relatively common terms, but other circumstances of baby loss are little talked about and may be unfamiliar. If you have never heard the term, you might not understand that ectopic pregnancy is a form of baby loss, for example. Similarly, unsuccessful conception might be considered sad and unfortunate, but not recognised as an experience of baby loss.

Different experiences of baby loss

Neonatal loss

Neonatal loss is the loss of a baby within the first 28 days of their life. Most neonatal loss is linked to premature birth, but some babies born at full term also have health complications which mean that they will not survive. The three main reasons for neonatal death are genetic disorders, a complication, or multiple complications, either during or after the birth, and infections. Some parents may know that their baby will face complications once they are born, while for others it only becomes clear when the baby arrives.

Neonatal care is the type of care that a baby born prematurely or with a medical condition receives. This is usually within a neonatal unit in a local hospital, but can sometimes be at a specialist hospital such as Great Ormond Street. If your baby is likely to require neonatal care, or to be cared for in a NICU (neonatal intensive care unit) when they are born, you can talk in detail with your midwife about where your baby will be cared for, what care they will need and how you can best prepare for some of the procedures. You might also have family members or a doula helping you prepare for the birth, and spending time talking about your fears and hopes, and grief about healthier outcomes that may already be present, can be part of your experience. Preparing for life with a newborn in neonatal care can be really challenging, especially if you have previously experienced baby loss. At a time when you hoped to be celebrating and sharing joy, you may be faced with having to understand a lot about a particular medical condition. Each person facing a period of neonatal care for their baby will handle it differently. You may want to know every detail of your baby's medical needs, or you may choose to ask your caregivers to only share certain details with you, while sharing other information with your partner or family. Making sure that you are honest about how you feel and allowing yourself to be sad about the situation is okay: you can and should still feel dignified and in charge of your choices.

Neonatal care for your baby does not always mean that you are going to experience baby loss. Every year in the UK neonatal care teams work extremely hard to ensure that they provide lifesaving medical support to the babies in their care. Many of the caregivers, neonatal nurses, doctors, and specialists are extraordinary people, with outstanding levels of compassion and expertise. Remember that they are there for you and for your baby, and that you can ask them any questions, make requests for the things that are important to you and your family and feel confident that they will hold you and your baby with genuine care. Sometimes, when your newborn needs a long stint of neonatal care, particularly if this includes separation from you with little or no touch, there can be grief for the loss of your initial time with your baby. Even if the outcome is that you eventually return home with your baby, there can be a sense of loss of the fourth trimester, when natural bonding and attachment was disrupted. You may have had to change your feeding routine to adapt to the needs of your baby, and while breastfeeding should be encouraged and supported wherever it is chosen and possible, there may be a difference between what your mind and body desire and what is physically possible for your baby. Professor Amy Brown of Swansea University has shown that grief and trauma can and do arise when breastfeeding doesn't work out as planned, so this may be another source of distress with which you will need support and time to heal.

Case study: neonatal loss

Noah was born at 37 weeks 6 days gestation by elective caesarean section. His parents Suzie and Andy already knew that he would be a very poorly baby. Noah had hyperplastic left heart condition, as well as a substantial number of additional complications. When Noah was 12 days old Suzie and Andy heard that he had Mosaic Patau's, a serious and rare genetic disorder, and it was at this point they knew that they would have to say goodbye to their baby. After 14 days of intense interventions, surgeries, and complex decisions about how to best care for Noah, he died in his mother's arms shortly after his first and final milk from her breast. Suzie was, at the time of Noah's death, also caring for her dying mother and very shortly after his funeral she became her mother's full-time carer, eventually moving into a hospice with her and her sister. While in the hospice Suzie and her sister surrounded their mother with love as she was cared for in the final weeks of her life. Reflecting with Suzie about her combined grief a year after Noah's passing and the subsequent loss of her mother, she spoke of the darkness she had and still did experience. 'Baby loss isn't clean sadness, is it?' she said 'It's not sit down and have a cup of tea sadness, that'll feel better once you have had a good chat about it, it is messy, dark, angry sadness. It is the sort of sadness that makes you want to hurt yourself and those feelings are not the sort of feelings that you want to share with anybody. When many of your friends are also mothers, you do not want to talk to them about the details of losing a baby, about the torturous detailed memories that keep coming back to mind'. In listening to Suzie and knowing her journey with Noah I have an awareness of just how much medical terminology, understanding and knowledge she and Andy had to get their heads around in an extremely short period of time. In those early days of caring for your newborn baby, when everything in a mother's body is hormonally and physiologically primed for feeding and holding and caring for your child, to have to become medical experts and key decision-makers about which procedures to follow, and how to manage the physical pain that your baby is in, requires a resilience and strength that is both admirable and deeply unfair. Suzie said 'The pain of the hope was unbearable, one day we thought he was doing well and was going to live and come home with us, the next day we were preparing to say goodbye'. Suzie is pregnant for the eighth time now, and her third baby is due later this year. She thinks of herself as a mother to three children: Arty who is three, Noah and the baby she is carrying. 'It is actually Andy who has really helped me with insight into how I understand the other losses', she says. Suzie has had two ectopic pregnancies, two miscarriages and a medical termination in and around the birth of her children. 'The way I see it is that my DNA, my mother's DNA, all of us are part of the same thing. My other losses were the loss of hope for a baby, but I have three children, and they are the ones that had and have potential for life and that potential, for every baby, for every child, is so fragile.'

Stillbirth

Stillbirth is when a baby dies at or after 24 weeks of pregnancy. In England one in every 200 births is a stillbirth. Sometimes a stillbirth might happen because of complications with the placenta, or it may occur for reasons which are never identified. Stillbirths may be identified by a routine scan, the mother experiencing physical pain or bleeding, or the onset of early labour. Many women find out that their baby will be stillborn when no heartbeat can be detected at an antenatal appointment, and for some the death of their baby happens during labour or birth.

If a baby has died, waiting for labour to start naturally or inducing labour are the preferred courses of action, depending on both choice and whether there are specific health concerns for the mother. It is very rare that a stillborn baby is born by caesarean section, as a physiological birth is deemed safer for women as the recovery carries less risk. Giving birth to a baby who has died can be very different to the birth of a live baby. Midwives and health professionals should give information and support to help prepare families for what to expect during labour, delivery and when the baby is born. Most hospitals have dedicated rooms away from other expectant parents and some have a specialist bereavement team to oversee care for families, especially if they are implementing the National Bereavement Care Pathway (see p54).

Case study: stillbirth

Luna's mum and dad were at home when they found out that their little girl had no heartbeat, during a routine check by a community midwife. This was then confirmed by two scans in hospital and mum's labour began within minutes of the confirmed absence of a heartbeat. A two-day labour brought their daughter into the world. Her birth was incredibly hard work, both physically and emotionally, ending in an assisted forceps delivery in theatre, but it was not without laughter and beauty. Mum was incredible, strong, and resilient and was accompanied by her partner, mother and me as their doula. The arrival of their daughter was beautiful and utterly devastating.

Mum spoke to me about the painfully lonely time of postnatal recovery after giving birth to Luna. The family was never visited by a health visitor, which is something they feel would have been supportive. Mum had difficulty accessing local bereavement/mental health support, and eventually sought private support from a counsellor.

In the early days after Luna died all I wanted to do was speak about my baby and about what was happening to my body. Others struggled to face this reality with me, and I found the only thing that really helped was the peer support we found through the SANDS charity. Their telephone support and group meetings. One of the most profound moments was when I first called the SANDS helpline, the first words of the lady who answered were 'Would you like to tell me about your baby?' This question had a deep and meaningful resonance for me and it is no surprise that the phone lines are run exclusively by parents who have lost babies at some stage in their lives. The physical meetings brought hope to the shadows for both me and my partner. Hearing stories from others who have also experienced baby loss, you are liberated by the honest exchange of your experiences. When conversing with those who haven't experienced baby loss, you often have to hold the space and carry the listener's empathy while they often 'imagine' the experience through the loss of their own children or loved ones. This becomes exhausting.

Mum reflected on Luna's birth with me recently, five weeks after the birth of her second daughter Maya. We spoke about how she felt then and how the arrival of Maya had been for her.

I feel that she has brought a huge amount of healing, I miss Luna now in a very different way than before. My body aches for her less now. I was really worried that when Maya arrived, I would be transported back to when we lost Luna, but that isn't what happened, I mostly just saw Maya.

I am aware that this is not the case for all families and when people suggested after Luna died that I would be able to try again, I was very angered by the idea that they thought I could replace Luna with another child. When you lose a child there is no happy ending. You must learn to live with the sadness and if you're lucky those around you support you in remembering your child. Maya is not a replacement for Luna, she is my second daughter and I am fortunate that for me, her arrival has been incredibly healing and has taken away some of the pain. Baby loss matters because it has a lasting impact on the lives of parents, their families and friends. It is not something we 'get over' or 'move on' from. We learn to live with the reality. In order to support women and families through loss we must open up a space for them to speak openly of their experiences and remember their children as they grow older. Baby loss is a taboo that brings shame and isolation. Together we must break the silence by sharing our stories and our children.

As a doula I was profoundly impacted by Luna's birth. She has informed my work and I am eternally grateful to her for her impact on my life.

Loss of healthier outcome

Sometimes, knowingly or unknowingly, we give birth to a baby who has a health condition, disability or syndrome which means that we must alter the way in which we care for them. This can sometimes include having to attend medical appointments, make adaptations to our homes or shift our expectations of daily family life. Having a baby with additional needs or with a specific health condition does not mean that your joy or delight in them should be compromised in any way, but for some people there can be a sense of loss of the healthier outcomes you had hoped for. In a beautifully diverse world, we all have unique and different bodies and celebrating your new family is an important part of your transition into parenthood, whether for the first time or as a sibling to your existing children. For some women and their families, however, there is also grief and loss that comes with the birth of a baby with additional needs. Loss of a healthier outcome is a very real experience for some, and it can be confused by those around them with not caring for or wanting the baby that they have. The shame that can be projected onto people in this situation can be all-consuming and lead to mental ill-health, postnatal depression, anxiety or isolation. Ensuring that we recognise that these people have also lost something that they anticipated for the future of their baby is important. Ensuring that access to appropriate psychological support is available can make all the difference to their recovery. It can be extremely isolating bringing up a baby that does not have the same ability as others, and it can be a hard adjustment for siblings to adapt to the routines required for their brother or sister's care. The groups and support networks that you anticipated joining may no longer be accessible or suitable, and you may feel isolated by your baby's care needs. It may feel like quite a leap to see this as baby loss, particularly if you have faced this in your own family and felt differently. As the grandparent, aunt, uncle or parent of a baby who is seemingly being considered as other than perfect by somebody else you may feel resentment or sadness, possibly even angry at the sense of loss felt by somebody else. All these feelings have value: they are all real and require deep empathy to support.

Case study: loss of healthier outcome

Rachel and Tom had baby Elsa in 2008. Rachel's pregnancy was smooth and Elsa was their third child. Soon after her birth Elsa began to show signs of auditory complications and it was soon found that she had severe hearing loss in both ears. Rachel said:

I was devastated. Here was my beautiful baby, the completion of our family, and she couldn't hear me. I remember coming home from the second screening test, armed with leaflets and advice from our audiologist and just thinking 'No – this isn't the baby I wanted' and then immediately feeling such a huge amount of guilt and shame that I didn't love my baby for who she was.

Tom felt quite differently about the discovery:

I was obviously concerned about Elsa, but I have worked to support people with disabilities and I just thought that we would find a way. It was hard for the first year, because I really wanted Rach to feel love and excitement for raising Elsa, but I could see that she was sad, almost grieving and that made the first year really hard for all of us. It wasn't her fault, but it has been hard for the two of us to reflect on that year as we look back.

Rachel realised that she felt as though she had experienced the loss of the baby that she had imagined, and shared with me some of the pain that she has felt.

> *You can't not love your baby, can you? I mean, I had a baby. I had a gorgeous, pretty, healthy baby and growing up deaf is not a bad thing. But I had imagined something different and I realise now that I had to grieve for the child that I had hoped I would have. I had to let go and learn a new set of expectations. The guilt that I felt in those first few years was really painful and I just remember feeling so lonely. Being part of the Deaf Mums group has saved me, meeting my new friends and realising that other people felt the same was really what got me through. And being really honest about what I was feeling, I could have tried to cover it up but by being honest I have been able to build a new relationship with the wonderful child that I have and my life is richer for being really honest about my grief and expectations.*

Stepparent baby loss

Becoming a stepparent to a baby can be challenging, not least because the intimate relationship with your partner may be new and may come straight off the back of a previous relationship for your new partner. In the early days of a new relationship having the additional responsibility of caring for your partner's baby, in whatever capacity you have agreed is right for you all, can put additional strain on your intimate and domestic life. While this may sound like a rare occurrence, it is surprising how often I hear stories of people experiencing the grief of baby loss in this way. This occurs when a new relationship starts shortly after the birth or conception of one partner's baby, either from a previous relationship or from a conception outside of a relationship, and the new partner adopts the role of stepparent to the baby. I have seen this happen really well, with amicable roles agreed between all of the parents, and I have seen it happen really badly, with individuals feeling that they had little choice but to assume the role of stepparent due to the way in which they have been allocated caring responsibilities. It is when the new relationship ends, or when previous arrangements change, that the new partner can experience baby loss.

The invisibility of this circumstance of loss is profound. Often the baby loss is not because of a baby dying, but happens because of a relationship ending. Navigating the unpredictable waves of grief that can occur as a stepparent is lonely and often overlooked by those around us.

Case study: stepparent baby loss

Neil and Chloe separated while she was pregnant with their first child. Chloe was already a mother to two older children and while the separation was amicable, Neil went on to start a new relationship with Sarah very soon afterwards. Sarah knew that within six months of moving in with Neil he would be sharing the care of his new baby with his ex. They agreed that while the baby was in his care, she would also be responsible for some of the baby's needs. At times she would be responsible for picking up the baby from Chloe while Neil was at work, and there would be occasions when the baby was in her sole care overnight. Sarah and baby Zaf inevitably became very close. She enjoyed and looked forward to her time as a stepparent and the relationships between all three of Zaf's parents were, for the most part, very healthy. When baby Zaf was eight months old Sarah experienced an early miscarriage.

I knew I wanted a child of my own biologically and when I found out I was pregnant I was really so happy. Having Zaf had shown me a side of myself that I always knew I wanted, to mother and to have a family.

Unfortunately, Neil and Sarah experienced a lot of challenges after her miscarriage and soon after they also separated.

I lost everything, not only my own baby, but my partner and Zaf when that happened. I went from seeing him every day, changing him, feeding him and putting him to sleep to just never seeing him. I went from having a future family to being totally alone, and the worst part was that it was all so invisible. My friends didn't know I had lost a baby and they hadn't really seen me with Zaf, so nobody apart from me thought of me as a mother.

Sarah explained that she did not know what to call herself, did not know how to reach out to people in a similar situation, and felt extremely alone in her grief.

I had imagined a life with my two children and knowing that one of them went on to live a life without me, well, the pain has never really left. I am doing other things now and try to remind myself that I still have those opportunities ahead of me, but I feel sad for the way this happens to people.

Forcible removal of a baby/traumatic separation

There are varying circumstances that can lead to a woman having her baby forcibly removed from her care. Babies born to women with issues related to substance misuse, in prison or living at risk of violence or harm to the newborn can and have faced circumstances whereby they are forced by law to give their baby into the care of another. In all circumstances of known pregnancy in which there is known risk to the unborn baby's safety, a thorough pre-birth assessment will be undertaken to identify the risks associated with family and environment, parenting capacity and the risk to the unborn baby. Official guidance on safeguarding unborn and newborn babies states:

> *If the conclusion of the pre-birth assessment is the baby cannot be adequately safeguarded in the parent(s) care, an Initial Child Protection Conference must be held to determine if the baby is at risk of significant harm when born and plan appropriate support and interventions, which may include the need to separate the baby from its mother. This can be a traumatic experience for the family and needs to be carried out sensitively with clear planning in place to assist all practitioners involved in undertaking their responsibilities.* Safeguarding Children Partnership

Removing a baby from their mother's care is rare, and not all forcible removals are permanent. Sometimes a woman may be supported to recover or change her circumstances and be reunited with her child. However, the separation of a baby from their mother shortly after birth will inevitably lead to traumatic grief from baby loss. Bereavement care and therapeutic care are provided to support emotional wellbeing and prevent further removals. It is vitally important that we work to ensure that women who have had to experience the devastation of having their baby removed from their care are still treated with respect and compassion. As birth workers we need to be prepared to meet women who have experienced this form of loss and hold space for them to approach future pregnancies with an awareness of the triggers and grief that may still be present for them. It is unlikely that you will just happen across this form of support in your role as a doula or midwife, as most situations requiring this level of support are handled by specialist organisations, charities or services. Birth workers engaged in supporting women who experience the removal of their baby should receive proper support, mentoring and guidance themselves.

Two police officers were present on the labour ward while she gave birth and although they weren't allowed in the room, every time I went to get my client ice, I had to walk past them. Knowing that within a few hours my client would have birthed and lost her baby was just terrifying. She was strong in labour and very quiet. Afterwards she spent four hours with her newborn girl, before being asked to sign the final documents required and give her baby over to the social worker who had been supporting her case. There are not the words to complete this story, she had her heart ripped away from her body and her eyes were blank, they took her heart away and as I sat there, comforting her body and holding her in the silence, I felt the terror of loss in the most profound and painful way imaginable – it was like being in hell. Anonymous birth companion

Miscarriage

Miscarriage is the most common kind of pregnancy loss. One in four pregnancies ends in miscarriage. A miscarriage is when a baby (or foetus or embryo) dies in the uterus during pregnancy. In the UK miscarriage is defined in pregnancies up to 23 weeks and six days gestation. After 24 weeks' gestation babies that die before birth are defined as stillbirths, while a baby that is born and lives for any amount of time and then dies will be defined as a live birth and neonatal death.

There are many different reasons why miscarriage occurs, and many are never understood or medically explained. Some of the reasons include anatomical complications for the mother, infection, or hormonal or genetic complications. Sometimes women can experience a miscarriage before they find out that they were pregnant and statistically most miscarriages occur in the first 12–13 weeks of pregnancy.

Sometimes a miscarriage will be identified at a routine scan, and this is referred to as a 'missed miscarriage'. There was nothing to indicate miscarriage prior to the scan. More commonly women will begin to experience symptoms such as spotting (leaking a small amount of blood), pain in the uterus or abdomen, cramping or no longer feeling the symptoms of a pregnancy such as sickness and breast tenderness.

If you experience a miscarriage you may pass your baby or pregnancy at home, or you may be treated in hospital. If you have a miscarriage in your first trimester you can choose to wait for it to complete naturally and once your pain and/ or bleeding has stopped you may be offered another scan to ensure that your body has completed the miscarriage. Alternatively, you may be asked to take a home pregnancy test. You can choose to take medication to begin the passing of your pregnancy. You will be offered tablets, usually in the form of a pessary inserted into your vagina. In most circumstances you will be able to go home for the miscarriage to complete. Sometimes surgery is offered under either local or general anaesthetic, during which your pregnancy is removed by a suction device. Miscarriages that occur later in pregnancy are often experienced within hospital settings unless you have already completed the miscarriage at home. A miscarriage that happens after 14 weeks' gestation may be referred to as a second-trimester or mid-trimester loss. The terminology around gestation and miscarriage can be very upsetting, as some parents will struggle to think of their mid-trimester loss as a miscarriage. They may birth a very developed baby who is a fully formed, tiny person, and to call this miscarriage can feel like the wrong definition for the loss.

Many of the words associated with the medical process of having a miscarriage are confusing and distressing, with such a range of experience of miscarriage between week one and week 24. You may refer to your miscarriage as your baby, your pregnancy or your child, or you may prefer to use less relationship-defining words such as tissue, cells, or contents of your uterus. You may refer to your experience as the birth, the miscarriage, the loss or the surgery, or a combination of these. No words are right for everybody. If you are facing a miscarriage or experience one in the future it is important to remember that respectful care is still vital. You should continue to have dignity and choice, and be spoken to in words that are empathic. It is a sad truth that very few women receive follow-up care when they experience a miscarriage, because they are so common. But giving birth, or completing your miscarriage at home, can be really scary, cramping during miscarriage can feel as intense as the contractions of labour, and very little information is provided to women about what to expect, what they will see or how they should recover. Information about the process of early miscarriage tends to be in the form of written leaflets or a brief conversation with a health professional, and many miscarriages take place away from a hospital setting and in the privacy of home. As a doula I have supported many women while they miscarry their babies at home. Seeking the support of a birth worker at this time can be a huge comfort, as you have companionship and empathy, your practical needs are taken care of and you have space to grieve and feel looked after.

Having attended miscarriages which have been sad but empowered and woman-led, I want you to know that in the face of the devastation of your loss you are still able to create a space and environment for birth, loss and healing that resonates with and for you. Sara miscarried her baby at home.

After writing the letter I did a ritual ceremony, which involved me putting a plant in the Earth for the soul, with a ribbon of love tied around, and having a fire to let go of anything I felt I needed to at that time. I found the letter and ceremony really helped me to come to terms with losing the baby, to help with letting go, saying goodbye and moving on. What also really helped, in what felt like a dark place I was in, was having a birth doula/ worker, who is also a friend, whom I love and respect greatly, in my home and in my life. Kay was checking in with me, being emotionally available and supportive. The information she gave, which I didn't know about, regarding what was going on in my body hormonally and otherwise, really helped me to surrender and be with it all. Sara Carter

Loss of a multiple
When you are expecting multiples and experience the loss of one or more of your babies it is tragic and can be extremely

hard to come to terms with, especially as you may continue to be pregnant, or be caring for the surviving multiple/s. Unfortunately, stillbirth and miscarriage are slightly more likely when you are carrying multiples and it is for this reason that managed labour is offered to many women who are carrying more than one baby.

You may experience the loss of one of your multiples early in your pregnancy and continue to carry all your babies to term or until a managed labour is deemed safe. This can be an emotional rollercoaster for women who must navigate the continuation of their live pregnancy with the knowledge that they are carrying one of their babies after loss. The loss of a twin during the first trimester of pregnancy does not usually affect the development of the surviving baby. With the loss of a twin in the second or third trimester, complications with the surviving twin are more likely, so your doctor will carefully monitor you and your baby. Some parents face the turmoil of selective reduction of risk, which means agreeing to the loss of one to save others.

Parents who have experienced the loss of a multiple face a life with a potentially lost identity for their babies and their own invisible knowledge of their sibling. Parents of triplets who birth two live babies may forever be asked about their twins, when they know that they have triplets. Comments such as 'Oh, but at least you have the other two' give no weight to the parents' grief for the baby lost.

They are my triplets, not my twins. As the years have gone by, every one of those moments is without their sister. I still see her. Daisy is there taking her first steps, saying her first words, she would probably have her first wobbly tooth now too. So, when people comment on my beautiful twin boys, my heart hurts for their sister, who

*walks alongside them every step of the way. We have
managed to keep Daisy alive in our hearts and lives, the
boys say goodnight to her at bedtime and sometimes she
is involved in their games, playing quietly alongside them.
They each have a Daisy cuddly toy and at night when I
walk in to tuck them into bed, if they are holding their
'Daisy toy' I am comforted by her continued presence.
I really wanted a daughter, a female companion in this
house of five men! She lives in my heart and every day
it breaks and mends, breaks and mends, over and over.*
Marie, mother to Daisy

There are fantastic charities and support services for
people who have experienced the loss of a multiple. Meeting
other parents who also have live children, while living with
the grief experienced after the loss of their sibling, can be
comforting, and they will understand your need to talk about
your missing baby/babies. The tacit expectation from others
that you should be grateful for what you have, and not grieve
for your baby loss, can lead to the reality of your grief being
quashed and invalidated. Support from those who understand
can be vital.

Molar pregnancy loss

Molar pregnancy, also known as hydatidiform mole, is a rare
complication of pregnancy in which there is an abnormal
growth of trophoblasts, the cells that normally develop into
the placenta. Molar pregnancies happen in two different ways:
complete molar pregnancy, and partial molar pregnancy. In a
complete molar pregnancy, the placental tissue is abnormal
and swollen and appears to form fluid-filled cysts. In a partial
molar pregnancy there may be normal placental tissue along

with abnormally forming placental tissue. There may also be formation of a foetus, but this is usually miscarried in early pregnancy. There are very few known cases of a baby surviving a molar pregnancy.

Approximately one in every 1,000 pregnancies is diagnosed as a molar pregnancy, and yet it is likely that many people will only hear about it when they or a friend experiences it. There can be many complications with molar pregnancy, as even after the loss and removal of the pregnancy, the molar tissue can continue to grow inside the womb. Sometimes this continued growth can lead to a type of cancer called choriocarcinoma, and facing the risk of cancer immediately or shortly after the loss of your pregnancy is extremely challenging and can be terrifying.

The consultant then took us to a small seating area curtained off from the scanner to talk through options. We opted for surgical management, as this pregnancy had clearly stopped progressing weeks ago but was not naturally miscarrying and with a little one at home I couldn't deal with the unknown of when or if it would happen. The consultant said something that will always stay with me 'You are allowed to grieve this loss, it is not just the loss of a pregnancy but the loss of what could have been, what you imagined this baby would be within your family, let yourselves grieve that too'. I spent the weekend mostly in tears, my mum offered to keep our little girl but I needed her close to cuddle in the middle of feeling such loss. I remember lying in bed with my hands on my tummy thinking to this little baby that I hoped they would hold on until Monday, that I wanted to cherish the small amount of time I still had with them being a part of me, even if they were already gone. I looked at the scan pictures of my little bean and you could see little arm and leg-like bumps sticking out. I cuddled my daughter and cried, went to bed and cried and talked with my husband and cried some more. During the months of testing I found hearing pregnancy announcements and seeing newborn babies really difficult, my baby should have been arriving in July but instead I was having bloods taken to watch out for cancerous growths. I still have the scan pictures about and look at them alongside the pictures from the early and booking scans for my next pregnancy with my son. It's now five years on and I can still see the expressions on the faces of the midwives and consultants, could still pick out which chairs we sat on in each waiting room and still feel that deep sense of loss when I think about that little bean-shaped blob on the screen just laying at the bottom of my womb but never moving. Emma Fraser

Ectopic pregnancy

An ectopic pregnancy is when a fertilised egg implants itself outside of the womb, usually in one of the fallopian tubes. The fallopian tubes connect the ovaries to the womb. If an egg gets stuck in them, it will not develop into a baby and the continuation of the pregnancy would compromise your health. Unfortunately, it is not possible to save the pregnancy and it usually must be removed using medicine or an operation. In the UK, around one in every 90 pregnancies is ectopic. This is around 11,000 pregnancies a year.

Alongside the loss of your pregnancy or baby you may also experience surgery which leads to the loss of your fallopian tube. In some cases, both fallopian tubes are removed. For many women this reduces the likelihood of future pregnancies and means they have to grieve not only their experience of the ectopic pregnancy, but also the lives ahead of them as biological mothers. However, there are options for future pregnancies, and many women do go on to have children after the removal of fallopian tubes, although the loss of 'natural' or 'conventional' routes to pregnancy is heartbreaking in itself.

Case study: ectopic pregnancy

Catherine experienced the loss of her pregnancy because of an ectopic pregnancy. She shared some of her insights into her experience and how her loss shaped her life afterwards.

Most of all I remember physical pain, emotional confusion, and dependence (on my parents, to help me). The ectopic changed the course of my life quite literally. When it happened, I was just on holiday in the UK but had been living in Spain for several years. As I couldn't travel for weeks, I had to stay with my parents and I lost my independence, couldn't work and began to reassess what my future was going to look like. Looking back, I think that the ectopic was the beginning of me having an entirely different life from the one that I imagined I would have. Before it, I used to think I would become a mother (when the time was right). After it, I went through different phases.

- *Initially (after the physical recovery part), I became terrified of sex because I thought I would have another ectopic (in the remaining fallopian tube) and die. This had an impact on relationships for quite a long time.*
- *Later (and as a single woman) I discovered that a new*

test had become available to find out whether the other fallopian tube was blocked too (it involves injecting dye). I went for this test alone – it was excruciatingly painful, and I could see from the nurse's reaction that the news was not good. I remember driving home alone, crying.

- *Next I was told that IVF would be the only option. I considered this but ultimately decided against it, for several reasons (not wanting motherhood to be such a medicalised process, going through it alone, having a friend going through it at the time and seeing how traumatic it could be…). So this was the point when I realised I was going to set out on a different, parallel path through life, and I began to accept that and make life good in other ways, through friendship and travel and work and the wider family and community.*

- *After a few more years, probably as I neared 40 and the biological imperatives had subsided, I actually began to feel liberated by not having had children. I suppose this was a time when I saw how exhausted and limited some of my friends, and my sister, felt by childcare and family life. During this time the friendships which strengthened for me tended to be those with others who didn't have children either. Looking back, I think I've lost three friendships because of the difficulties/misunderstandings of being parents or not.*

- *Despite the process of acceptance and a general sense of being at peace with life as it is, there are sometimes moments which take me by surprise, such as a friend's son turning 18 around the time I might have been celebrating a child's 18th, or when friends become or talk about becoming grandparents…* Catherine

Ectopic pregnancy is rarely spoken about, with many people referring to their loss as a miscarriage or early pregnancy loss, and the silence around living life with one or no fallopian tubes is very evident. The loss of parts of your body, which were vital to your expectation for parenthood, brings its own grief. This was true for Phillipa when she experienced the loss of her fallopian tubes during her pregnancy earlier this year:

8.30pm was when I went down for surgery. Being taken down to the surgical room was the most overwhelming thing I have ever experienced. I was awake while the team prepared the room, their equipment and themselves. I felt like I had been given a sentence for something criminal and being punished for something I hadn't done – an injustice of some sort. Not for one second did I appreciate this was saving my life – all I wanted was for our pea to be in the right pod, its rightful pod – my womb – and for us to go home.

The 'what ifs' are the worst thing about having to deal with life after our pregnancy loss. The 'What if our pea made it to its pod?', the 'Would our pea have carried on growing if they made it to my womb?', the 'What if I didn't make that call to the GP?', the 'What if my GP was so consumed by COVID and didn't realise my concerns?', the 'What if I ended up having lifesaving surgery', the 'What if I died?'. But the main one for me, as I can't speak on behalf of Conor, is the 'What if this wasn't supposed to be our journey and we were able to naturally conceive?'. We now won't be able to do that, the one time we managed it wasn't viable, and we lost our pea and remaining tube.

I can no longer accept that this happened for a reason and it wasn't meant to be, it doesn't offer comfort at times

*of devastating pain. I will accept there is no reason for
such a loss but our loss is the reason why we loved you –
our should-have-been baby!* Phillipa Choong

Abortion/termination of pregnancy

Baby or pregnancy loss which happens as the result of a
termination is a very complex issue. It is the elephant in the
room of our silent relationship to baby loss, and the one
circumstance of loss that I adamantly insisted was included
in this conversation and book. With all my heart I want to
stand with you and offer my conviction that baby loss and
pregnancy loss absolutely can happen when you face the
decision as to whether or not to have a termination. While pro-
life campaigners worldwide continue to shout loud messages
to the contrary, there is nothing within your experience of
a termination or abortion of pregnancy that separates you
from having a right to grief. You may come to the decision
to terminate your pregnancy without having any desire to
parent and an interpretation of your experience as baby loss
may not be right for you at all. If you experience an abortion
and do not feel that you have lost a baby, that is completely
fine and you may find relief in the end of your pregnancy,
move on with your life and find peace in the certainty of your
decision. There are seven different grounds for termination
of a pregnancy in Britain, according to the Abortion Act.
These are described in the Royal College of Obstetricians and
Gynaecologists clinical guidelines as follows:

*Abortion is legal in Great Britain if two doctors decide
in good faith that in relation to a pregnancy one or more
of the grounds specified in the Abortion Act are met (1).*

A *The continuance of the pregnancy would involve risk to the life of the pregnant woman greater than if the pregnancy were terminated.*

B *The termination is necessary to prevent grave permanent injury to the physical or mental health of the pregnant woman.*

C *The pregnancy has not exceeded its 24th week and the continuance of the pregnancy would involve risk, greater than if the pregnancy were terminated, of injury to the physical or mental health of the pregnant woman.*

D *The pregnancy has not exceeded its 24th week and the continuance of the pregnancy would involve risk, greater than if the pregnancy were terminated, of injury to the physical or mental health of any existing child(ren) of the family of the pregnant woman.*

E *There is a substantial risk that if the child were born it would suffer from such physical or mental abnormalities as to be seriously handicapped. The Act also permits abortion to be performed in an emergency if a doctor is of the opinion formed in good faith that termination is immediately necessary.*

F *To save the life of the pregnant woman.*

G *To prevent grave permanent injury to the physical or mental health of the pregnant woman.*

Most terminations carried out in England are carried out under ground C. In 2018, there were 205,295 abortions in England and Wales. The abortion rate was highest for those aged 21, and 81 percent of those women were single. There are a lot of single, young people going through the possibility of deep grief, with the additional vulnerability of societal shaming, blame and misunderstanding. Unless you have been informed by a woman who has experienced a termination that she does not have grief about her loss, it is worthwhile offering her compassion rather than judgement. This may require you to put aside your personal beliefs, opinions and experiences.

Parents faced with having to undergo terminations on other grounds will have to endure the devastation of giving consent to 'termination of pregnancy', to use the medical terminology. To have to sign away the much hoped-for life of your child is not something anyone should have to do, and while many terminations have saved women from fatalities and health complications for them and their baby, it may seem against the natural order of what you had come to expect and hoped for. That you have had to give 'consent' for the procedure, which is societally shrouded in blame and guilt, is hugely unfair. That your grief may be viewed by people as your fault – as your choice – is not okay.

Undergoing a termination is not easy, enjoyable, or relieving: it is hard work and can be painful both physically and emotionally, even if the termination is very much desired. During terminations women can be triggered by previous circumstances of loss, by the conditions of their current or historic relationships and by the judgement of others. If these women come to identify as having experienced the loss of a baby or pregnancy, or the loss of part of themselves or their identity, we must strive to ensure that their grief and loss is acknowledged and held with grace and compassion.

Knowing that I had to sign a form to have my baby terminated from me was devastating. Like I had a choice, like by signing that form I was willing. I was not. My baby was wanted – my pregnancy was wanted. I felt like I was being tortured and lying when I put pen to paper. NO, it is not okay for you to terminate my pregnancy, NO! But what else can you do? Why they can't call it

something different I don't understand. I have told two
people that I terminated my pregnancy, others I tell that
I lost my baby, because I can't face the judgement of it. At
school there was a girl who had an abortion and I know
what people thought about her, I wasn't going to have
people think the same about me. So mostly I don't even
talk about it. It was four years ago, and when I think that
I could have a four-year-old child I just feel so confused
still about why nobody ever really thinks to ask me about
her. I have a box with my scan picture, a cute little rattle
thing that my Mum gave me from my Grandma and the
hospital band that I wore when I was in. That's it, that is
the sum total of what I am allowed to remember from my
role as a Mum. Anonymous, mother to D

If you have experienced loss and have grief resulting from a
pregnancy or baby that was terminated, on whatever grounds,
in whatever circumstance, I see you. You are allowed to grieve
for this life. You can be very sad about the decisions that you
had to make, and you are absolutely allowed to miss your baby.

Premature baby loss

Premature labour is labour that happens before the 37th week
of pregnancy. According to leading premature baby research
charity Borne, prematurity is the leading cause of death in
newborn babies. In the UK, one in 13 babies are born preterm
and 60,000 families are affected every year. More significant
than infection, trauma or cancer, premature birth affects
some 15 million babies across the world each year. One in
10 premature babies are permanently disabled.

If you have experienced the premature birth of your baby,
you are very likely to have also spent some time visiting them
in neonatal care. Your time with your baby may have been very

short, and for some families it may have been several weeks or months of visits to your NICU (neonatal intensive care unit). In NICU you meet other families and babies and are exposed to many experiences of loss all at once. Not only are you deeply within your own grief, but the NICU can also be associated with other people's stories and experiences of loss, and you may have lived your life after birth in a continuous cycle of hope and loss. Life inside a NICU unit can be extremely hard on parents, who have to adjust to the medical information and the noise of the breathing machines, and the turmoil of seeing other families come and go, sometimes with a baby and sometimes without.

One of the challenges of having a baby in intensive care is repeatedly having to go home without your baby. Your loss may have been extended over a very long period, and your mental health may have suffered from the continuous cycle of 'what ifs'. Parents who have shared their stories of premature loss of their baby have reflected on the increased anxiety that has stayed with them ever since.

It is also possible that in the midst of your grief you will meet other parents in NICU who become your support network as you grieve together and fully understand what you have been through together. This will not lessen your loss, but may be of comfort in your grief.

She was so tiny at first, not even really like a baby. I just assumed that she was dead and then when the doctors all started to rush around, and she was gone I suddenly realised that she was alive, and they were trying to save her. It was impossible to think that somebody so small could be alive. Every day was hard, coming home without her day in, day out, going to work, meeting up with friends and trying to do normal life, except our life wasn't normal, the normal we were expecting was to have her at home and she wasn't there. And then that dreaded morning just as we were setting off to visit her and they called, and we knew and we just fell apart – it was earth-shattering. We had been going to her every day for six weeks and now she was gone. Shaih, father to Emma

Loss due to infertility or fertility-related issues

Infertility is the inability to reproduce by natural means. Fertility issues span a wide range of possible complications, diseases, genetic disorders, hormonal challenges, and previous baby loss circumstances, all of which result in the need for you to seek assistance in getting pregnant. For some women and birthing people and their partners (where one is involved) there are relatively simple solutions to overcoming fertility issues, while for others it may take several rounds of treatment. The broad term for such treatment is 'assisted reproduction'.

Assisted reproduction includes but is not limited to:

- IVF (*in vitro* fertilisation), in which an egg is sourced from the woman's ovaries and fertilised with sperm in a laboratory. The fertilised egg, called an embryo, is returned to the womb to develop.
- IUI (intrauterine insemination), a type of artificial insemination in which sperm is placed inside the womb.
- and ICI (intracervical insemination), where sperm is placed at the cervix (the neck of the womb).

Assisted reproduction can also happen with the use of donor sperm (donor insemination) or eggs (egg donation).

There are many different routes to overcoming fertility issues and you can find further information in the resources section at the end of the book. The availability of options is ever-increasing and so are the rates of success. However, for some the path to conception is far from easy, and in the words of fertility writer, speaker and blogger Katy Lindemann, '*You live in a cycle of hope and hopelessness. Hope can be cruel.*' If you have experienced baby loss as a result of fertility issues which cannot be overcome, or if you have come to the end of your journey with attempted conception, your grief can be heartbreaking and despairing, and be coupled with the weight of grief for a healthier or more fertile body.

Assisted reproduction is often silenced and hidden, and many spend weeks or years on an almost invisible journey of attempting conception. When these people choose to share with others they are often met with persistent and seemingly dismissive offers of resilience and hope, as people encourage them 'not to give up', or promise 'You'll get there eventually'. But unless we are fertility experts, we cannot ever be the voice of authority on individual circumstances. We wish our family, friends, clients, and colleagues well, but a persistent message of 'keep hoping' can be detrimental when not offered with an awareness of grief that may be present.

Infertility grief

Naava Carman is a traditional Chinese medicine acupuncturist and herbalist who has specialised in treating female and male fertility, gynaecology and obstetrics for over 20 years. She is focused on women who are 38–45 years old with complex, multifaceted fertility issues, such as autoimmune disorders, unexplained infertility, failed IVF, recurrent miscarriage, hypermobility, PCOS, endometriosis and other inflammatory conditions. www.fertilitysupport.co.uk

Infertility grief sits in a space all on its own. It's a delicate thing to talk about with my clients, who often open up about their feelings with much caveating and comparing.

'It's not the same as if I'd miscarried.'

'It's not the same as if I had a baby who died.'

'It's not the same as if I had a child who died.'

Here's the thing: nobody is saying it is the same. It's different, and it is no less important a journey to honour. If we use comparison as a tool for allowing emotions to be validated, then we would all be stuck in trauma. That is often where my clients are when they first come to see me. They've been on a long, unrewarding, relationship-sapping rollercoaster with no end in sight. They feel powerless, angry, sad, full of grief – and unable to express this for fear of taking up space on the grief spectrum to which they don't feel they can lay a rightful claim.

Losing a baby or child is 'out there' – it is accepted grief, and it isn't a grief that anyone is expected to get over quickly. Everyone understands if it is therefore hard for the client to be around children, nobody asks when they might try again, and nobody suggests that they stop trying for a family if it is too hard. These, however, are things which regularly get said to my clients, and combined with a level of necessary privacy most people feel they are quite rightly due when they are trying for a family, this is a layer of pressure and expectation which allows little to no space for grief to be present.

Every time a client tries to conceive, they feel hope and they begin to imagine a possible future. Each time their period arrives, that hope is dashed to the floor (all too often along with their self-image and happiness) and they have to pick themselves up, deal with their grief hitting them in the face again, and prepare to try anew.

Part of what a fertility acupuncturist does is to function as a detective. We understand the journey from both a western medical and traditional Chinese medicine point of view, and we can look at every aspect of it, from examinations and blood tests to operations to failed IVF cycles, and see what is missing, what needs to be done, who to go and see, and how long it will take. Inherent in this process is the premise that we need to help our clients regain a sense of control over their journey, that our support and compassionate presence alongside them allows them the space to express their feelings and be heard, and that our treatment allows clients to see a clear difference in symptoms and results, which lead to a better outcome.

Infertility grief is often silent, but it is real, and shouldn't be ignored or ultimately dealt with without external help and expert tools. Suffering alone for months or years is not necessary, but reaching out is often the hardest thing to do when the silence around this issue is so societally deafening. If someone is reading this piece who is sitting in grief, then I would encourage them to reach out to find a practitioner to vent to, to depend on, and who will validate their lived experience. Ultimately this grief has an ending, but sometimes someone like me needs to hold that knowledge, positivity and hope for their clients until they are ready to pick it up again themselves.

Sudden Infant Death

When a baby up the age of 12 months dies suddenly and their death is unexpected, there are a few different terms that are used to describe the loss. Most common are sudden unexpected death of infancy (SUDI) or sudden infant death syndrome (SIDS). You may have heard the term 'cot death' to describe the unexpected or sudden death of a baby. This term is still sometimes used, but it can be confusing because it suggests that the death of a baby is linked exclusively to their sleeping environment.

The Lullaby Trust provides vital support services for people and families who have experienced the sudden or unexpected death of their baby. Their guidance highlights that:

Some sudden and unexpected deaths can be explained by the post-mortem examination, revealing, for example, an unforeseen infection or metabolic disorder. Deaths that remain unexplained after the post-mortem are usually registered as 'sudden infant death syndrome' (SIDS) or 'sudden unexplained death in childhood' (SUDC) in a child over 12 months. Sometimes other terms such as SUDI (sudden unexpected death in infancy) or 'unascertained' may be used.

Case study: Sudden Infant Death

Sue is 72, a grandmother to five children and mother to three. Her second baby died unexpectedly at four months. Sue has shared some of her insight into how she has lived a life deeply affected by the loss of her baby.

Rosaline was a sweet child, my second. I remember her birth as vividly as I do the birth of my two other children, quite easy with all of them, I guess that was lucky, some don't have it easy do they? It was harder with two and I had Rosa when my son was still just running around my ankles. But then there was that god-awful day when I woke up to find my daughter lifeless next to me.

Sue experienced the loss of her baby over 45 years ago and when she shares her story of the day she woke up next to her daughter, who had unexpectedly died in the night, her emotions are still very raw and very real. The description of the shock that Sue and her husband experienced on that day is heartbreaking and frightening.

As I sat holding her to my chest, I wanted everything to end. I was howling and screaming, it was the scariest moment of my life. For many days afterwards I wanted everything to end. I wanted my baby girl back in my arms, I wanted to rewind time just those few hours to when I had settled her under her blanket. There was no explaining why she died, I will never have the answer to that.

Sue describes the first two years after the loss of her daughter as the hardest in her life. She has shared with me the challenges of raising her son, of learning of her third pregnancy and the journey she has been on to find peace, despite never feeling that she will ever fully heal from the loss of her first daughter.

People are what have brought me peace, kind and caring people, who have given me strength and kept Rosa alive in their memories. I have several friends who still even now, would you believe, send a card on her birthday or on the day that she died. To have people keep her spirit alive and remember me as her mother, whilst allowing me to be horribly awful to be around, that is love and friendship. I have my second daughter, which has brought me a lot of peace. It was hard at first but now my daughter is grown up and we have always remembered our angel Rosaline. We share photographs of her, and we say a blessing for her at special family events. She is still very present, and yet the pain of loss is, even now, something that is enormous to live with. The pain of loss and well, just the shock. The shock took longer to find peace with than the loss.

Sue has found comfort in sharing her experience with other women, and the strength that she feels that she has given to her second daughter.

I was there for the birth of two of my grandchildren and that was healing. My daughter looked into my eyes as she birthed my grandchildren, and in her eyes, I knew she drew strength from what she has seen me endure. That is a great gift to be able to give to your child, inspiration and evidence of how strong us women are. Despite the pain of it all, my Rosa gave me that strength.

Medical terminology and loss

Loss is often coupled with medical care, often in a hospital setting. While there are circumstances in which women and birthing people choose to freebirth and free miscarry (give birth, or pass pregnancy without medical support), it is not very common in cases of late pregnancy baby loss. The language used to describe what happens to us medically can add weight to the despair and grief that we feel when we hear of a loss of life. Many of the saddest moments come when women and their partners have to sign forms, or listen to information about their precious baby, which does not seem to capture, acknowledge or fit with the love, hope and life associated with the pregnancy.

A shift away from pain and towards compassion has to come from our caregivers. To hear your baby referred to in medical terms can be emotionally devastating, and unfortunately sometimes we have to sign consent forms that makes it sound as if we are willingly choosing our loss. As a birth worker I ask my clients to choose words that are most suitable for them, and while it is sometimes very rushed and in the midst of a medical emergency, if possible I encourage the use of a loss birth plan, which allows me and my clients to request that medical staff refer to the loss in words that are right for the client. If the baby has a name, I encourage medical staff to use it rather than using medical language. This is not always successful, and medical professionals who are not directly involved in maternity or midwifery struggle to adapt to referring to the 'removal of the products of pregnancy' by a name. Midwives and particularly bereavement midwives often have the most compassion, but unfortunately baby and pregnancy loss are not always supported exclusively by maternity staff, and sometimes health professionals from different departments, units or wards are involved, and they are duty-bound to ensure that they have clearly obtained consent and understanding, which explains their use of the 'correct' medical terms. However, there is a lot of scope for additional training around language and compassion, particularly in emergency situations within NHS care, and I appeal to all health professionals to examine how they communicate with parents experiencing shock, tragedy and loss.

I encourage you to continue to advocate for support wherever it is possible. If you notice one particular member of staff who appears more empathic, try to direct your questions to them, or recruit a loss doula or birth doula. If words are hurtful or cutting, always feel able to state the need for compassion. It is not your responsibility to seek compassion from medical staff, but it is your right to receive dignified and respectful care and if you are not then you can point that out.

The next day was sunny Good Friday, the beginning of the glorious Easter weekend. It started off being the worst day of my life. They had rushed me in for a scan first thing, to carry out an invasive procedure to confirm the assumed diagnosis. I went into the hospital alone as my partner was banished to the car (due to corona!). I met with a consultant who scanned me, confirmed that my little one had 'deformities consistent with trisomy 18' and then softly announced that my baby was a little girl. We had a frank conversation about her prognosis, and her unlikeliness to survive for much longer. The ultrasound findings were so severe that he offered to start the induction process of labour today. Just 24 hours before, I was pregnant and still had a sliver of belief that all would be okay. And here I was, surrounded by strangers in masks, signing a consent form headed 'termination for foetal abnormality incompatible with life'. Francine Bridge, mother to April

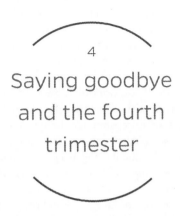

4

Saying goodbye and the fourth trimester

Meeting your baby

They popped her basket down on the bed next to me, and we just cried. There she was – translucent skin and big blue-black eyes looking right at us and she melted our hearts. In that moment it felt like the most natural thing. It did not matter that she wasn't fully grown. We both felt a sense of peace. She was here and she had done what she set out to do – whatever that was. Her role was fulfilled.
Christina Clarke, mother to Poppy

Describing what it is like to see and hold a baby who is not alive may feel devastatingly sad. Some women and birthing people and their partners choose not to see or hold their baby or pregnancy after it is complete, and this is entirely your choice. Even writing these words is hard. It is rare that we ever get to see a dead body, let alone that of our baby. And yet many parents have told me that they wish that they had known what to expect. Many women who I have spoken to about miscarriage were confused by what they were seeing, and unsure of what they were supposed to 'do' with their loss. If these words are too hard to read, please move on to the next section. For those of you working to support birth, especially if you have not experienced a loss before, I encourage you to read on. Having some preparation prior to your first experience of supporting loss is important: you can work to comfort and support your client without being in a state of shock yourself. It is also important to make clear that dead babies are completely beautiful. Beyond the signs of lifelessness are the delicate forms of each finger and toe, the little noses and cheeks, round bellies and soft hair. It may be different from what we are used to, but in so many ways it is perfect.

Not all baby loss will lead to a meeting with your baby. Often in early pregnancy loss, the foetus is so small that you may pass what looks like blood, mucus and clots. However, some women do see their baby even in early miscarriage, and it is possible that you will see and identify parts of your baby's body as you miscarry. Talking about what you see seems to carry even more taboo and is even more hidden than the experience itself. It may be that you meet your baby when you miscarry later in pregnancy, or when they are born stillborn. You may also come to baby loss after having a live birth.

Until I worked as a doula supporting loss, the only experience I had was supporting two friends through terminations and my own miscarriage. I remember studying my loss, looking for the features in among the blood, being terrified and flushing my miscarriage away, not wanting to look. And then I felt guilt. I had just flushed away my pregnancy, my baby. Absolutely nothing had prepared me for this. Nobody had described what I would or would not see, and I was in my bathroom alone and in quite a lot of pain.

When you meet a baby who is dead, they can look very different from a live baby. They may be very small, and have quite a translucent skin tone. Older babies may be fully formed, with all the details of their body intact. Some babies are born with dark lips, due to blood pooling or asphyxia. Your baby's skin may have begun to peel, and this might be slight or more advanced and look raw or missing in areas. Sometimes you may be able to see some of your baby's organs, and this can be distressing if you are not expecting it. Dead babies have no muscle tone and are limp to hold; they do not respond to any reflexes and will not be supporting themselves in any way. This can make it slightly tricky to handle your baby, as they are not responsive to your movement. Most babies born in hospital will be handed to you wrapped in a blanket, but you can request skin-to-skin contact if you are aware that your baby will be stillborn or a later miscarriage. In most circumstances when a stillbirth is discovered at birth your baby will be taken care of straight away by midwives or doctors, who may be trying to revive your baby or assess what is happening. Your baby's head may appear to be a different shape than a live baby's, with some experiencing skull collapse with overlapping cranial bones. Some are born with wide open mouths and eyes.

Some parents decide that they would like to take their baby home with them. This is legal and possible if a coroner has not ordered a postmortem. Your midwife will be able to provide you with information about meeting your baby, how you would like to do this and whether or not you want to hold your baby, leave them at hospital or take them home. If you are in hospital and choose not to see your baby at first, they will be kept in the hospital, and kept cold to slow the decline in skin quality and retain their appearance. If you decide that you would like to hold your baby a few hours or even days after you have given birth, this is possible. Your midwife can take a photograph of your baby or loss if you would rather not see them. You can choose to take these photographs home with you to look at when you are ready.

Nobody tells you that your baby will have black lips. Of course, I knew that my baby wouldn't look alive, but I just couldn't stop staring at her lips, black lips. The shock of holding her body, the looseness of her neck, the familiarity of her features, she was just like her sister, but she had black lips, and nobody told me that she would. There is something about all the hospital memorabilia, all the preciousness, the blue boxes, pink boxes, ribbons and footprints that just didn't make me feel better. My baby was not a pastel memory box, she was my future and she could not move, and her lips were black. Zara, mother to Esther

Meeting your baby is absolutely your choice and you should feel able to decide how it happens. I have witnessed parents find great joy holding and studying their baby after loss and I have also known women decide not to hold or see their baby. You are being asked to make a decision on something that is against all of your expectations, and if it is not right for you to meet your baby, please find comfort in knowing that this is okay. You are allowed to feel scared, nervous, distressed and unsure. Meeting your baby can be beautiful, peaceful, and healing, but for some it might feel the opposite. Allowing yourself to do what is right for you is important, as is taking a moment to consider how you might feel in the future. If you have a sense that you may regret not meeting your baby, it might feel possible to see them wrapped in a blanket in your midwife's arms. You may choose to just see their face, or their hands or feet. You may have close relatives who would like to meet and perhaps hold your baby. Again, this is led by you. If you are willing your midwife can support this, either in the same room as you, or in a room away from you. Your permission will have to be given for this to happen.

If you are giving birth as part of a couple one of you may choose to meet your baby and the other not. This can be challenging and you may feel that you are in disagreement – one stronger, one not, or one rejecting, one not. No two people are the same and the choices that you make have to be right for you. You cannot coerce somebody into meeting their baby if they do not want to. Having deep empathy for one another in these decisions will be of great benefit to you.

I feel that collectively the medical terminology used back then, the lack of information to hand with regard to 'missed' miscarriages, the feeling of the conveyor belt system, the subject and the fact that I was expected to keep this all to myself then played a huge part in the trauma felt. As I could not discuss it with my own mother and the dissociation from my partner, I felt there was no pathway for expression. I felt alone, lost and confused and as a result this had a major impact on my psyche, which I carried for 15 years. In hindsight I would have liked to have been given the option and choice to have access to my babies' foetuses, so that I could say goodbye in my own way, which would have helped with the process of acceptance. Lucy Wilson

If you experience baby loss at home, you can wrap your baby

or pregnancy loss in a blanket or towel and keep them close to you or in a safe space such as a crib or basket in your home until you have a medical professional with you to handle the next steps. After an early miscarriage at home, you may not need further medical support, in which case what you decide is right for your loss is up to you. If you would like to bury your baby you can, or if you would like to ask somebody to remove the loss and wrap it for you then that is fine. If you are unsure of what to do, contact the hospital and ask for their advice. You can also contact any of the loss charities listed in the resources section. In a medical emergency, you should always call 999.

You may choose to take some photographs of your baby or loss. This is completely fine, and how you choose to share or display these images is also fine. Many women have framed pictures of themselves holding their baby, and some create an announcement to share on social media or with friends. I encourage everyone to consider the impact of sharing images, and to be sensitive to the needs of people who have experienced trauma or previous loss. While I absolutely encourage you to share whatever feels right for you, placing an appropriate trigger warning at the beginning of any public-facing posts will allow people to choose to look away.

After cuddles, kisses, photos and gazing at her in awe, we handed her back over to the midwives just after midnight. A part of me felt bad that I wasn't choosing to spend overnight with her. But the truth was, I didn't want to grow too attached to having her and then go through the even greater heartache of handing her back over and leaving without her in the morning... I almost wanted the emotional goodbye to happen sooner rather than later. I feel guilty for thinking this but it's how I coped at the time. Francine Bridge, mother to April

Saying goodbye and remembering

Meeting your baby may be when you choose to say your final goodbye, or you may wish to consider a more ceremonial event or ritual to mark your loss. There are so many ways to do this and you may feel keen to do several, have a formal funeral or indeed to do nothing more than leave the hospital and go home. Most hospitals will offer you a range of options for keepsakes for your baby. You may request a lock of their hair, hand or footprints, their cord clamp or the blanket they were wrapped in. Some hospitals can store these keepsakes if you feel unable to take them home with you and some will provide you with a box or envelope in which these items can be sealed.

Having a funeral may feel right for you and you can talk to your midwife about the arrangements that you may need to make for this to happen. Some women choose to hold a traditional funeral, while others choose a ceremony that resonates with their beliefs, practices and personal choices. I have known couples to work alongside artists to create sand mandalas, paintings and pottery to acknowledge their baby's life, and there are many different keepsakes that you may wish to purchase or create.

My husband and I carried his wicker coffin through the church. We read poems and I spoke about our journey. We listened to music and my dad was amazing. We went to the pub and I laughed with friends and hugged them and felt the sunshine. But I knew something changed forever and that I had never known a sadness so consuming and deep. Lois Darcy, mother to Bodhi

Having a physical object to represent, remember, touch and hold can be of comfort. These objects can be a way to charge something physical with the energy that you have for your non-physical child. Potter and artist Rosie McLachlan explores the ways in which physical objects can be created as powerful memory-invokers:

Objects are powerful; they engage our emotions and invoke memories, ideas and meanings in our minds. Certain objects can be strongly associated with a loss we have experienced. These symbolic objects can help us to both grieve and celebrate a life. Not all experiences of loss have significant objects associated with them. Sometimes we are left empty-handed. If this is your experience, the act of finding or creating an object that represents your loss can be a powerful and healing thing.

The presence of a symbolic object is what makes it powerful. Part of the pain of loss is a feeling of profound absence. We can get lost in that empty space. An object that embodies your loss can reorient you, as focusing on it can help to break the seal of grief. This is because grief does not necessarily come on demand. It is something that must be evoked through stories and images.

As we grieve, at some point in time and space, an object that symbolises loss can transform into a symbol of love. It becomes a source of remembrance, a tangible representation of a life, and your love for that life. To live with a symbolic object is to experience a presence that will accompany you in the cycle of grieving and loving throughout your life.

You may choose to host a naming ceremony or grief ritual for your baby or loss. It might feel right to bury or burn the placenta, share stories, or read poetry or words. All these options can be decided after the initial event of loss and you must agree what feels right for you and your partner, family, and close relatives. It may be some time before you feel ready to host or hold any form of event, and whether you decide to delay for a few weeks, mark it on the anniversary of your loss or indeed never do anything, all of these choices are valid. It is also never too late. I recently attended a ceremony to say goodbye to a baby who was stillborn 20 years ago. The mother had never considered a funeral or ceremony at the time and she came to realise that it was important to her to say goodbye alongside her friends and family. During this sacred fire and circle, we gathered to release her baby from this world and to celebrate the recovery that had been found.

And I lay you to rest. Along with my grief, you take with you an irreplaceable piece of my heart and this will always be just yours. Sleep now my child, you are always remembered, always loved and have led me home to myself with your spirit. Sue, mother to C

The fourth trimester after loss

The fourth trimester is the time after your baby is born until they are three months old. More and more information is being offered through books, support groups, exercise classes and online to ensure that women and birthing people approach this important time with care and consideration for the changes in their bodies and lives. Unfortunately, much of this available support forgets to include those who are going through the fourth trimester without a baby. Where it is included, it tends to be in a sub-section entitled 'special circumstances', which is of course surrounded by chapters that focus on life with a baby. For many people affected by loss this makes the whole book or class, webpage or guidance sheet inaccessible because it is too painful to read. I encourage more birth workers to think about how they can ensure that information about the fourth trimester, postnatal recovery, labour and birth can be accessed by a parent or person who has experienced loss.

The timing of your loss will have a significant impact on how you experience the physical challenges of the fourth trimester. If you have experienced an early miscarriage, ectopic or molar pregnancy, or the early termination of your pregnancy, your body is likely to return to its pre-pregnancy condition relatively quickly. You will experience some bleeding and hormonal rebalancing, and it may take a while for your menstrual cycle to return to its normal pattern. This is not the case for all early cases of baby loss, and you may experience a significant fourth trimester after any circumstance of loss. For others, recovery from the loss of their baby or pregnancy also involves recovering from surgery that has altered their own body significantly. In the case of ectopic pregnancy, some molar pregnancies, emergency caesarean sections and hysterectomies you may be entering your fourth trimester healing from personal physical and emotional loss, as well as from baby loss.

Pregnancy is a physiological and endocrinological miracle, and even though we can scan bellies, perform lifesaving surgery and provide treatments and drugs to cure many illnesses we still have much to understand about gestation and birth. What your body did is truly incredible and it is no surprise that this alteration requires a period of readjustment. Hormonal changes begin very early in pregnancy. So although your pregnancy may have ended with the devastating loss of your baby, you may continue to experience physical changes for a long time afterwards. This stage of postnatal recovery, in situations of loss, can be isolating and confusing. There are very few groups for postnatal recovery after loss. While your friends access parenting groups, yoga classes, breastfeeding support groups, stay and plays and other community-focused services, you are suddenly alone, without a community on hand that you easily fit into.

My D+C was straightforward from a surgical perspective and my partner took me back to our hotel three hours post-op from recovery. We drove the four hours home the following day and I couldn't stop ruminating how it felt like my fault, like my body failed me and that I couldn't keep my baby safe. I had two weeks off work and ended up with endometritis from retained products and was totally miserable. My mental health suffered extremely those first few weeks before my genetic results came in and I was unable to leave my house or really function. I hadn't expected to have my milk come in five days post D+C due to my early gestation and found that extremely distressing. Kelsey Brumpton, mother to Jasper+3

Hormones

During pregnancy, your body produces an incredible cocktail of hormones, which you respond to both physically and emotionally. You will have increased follicle stimulating hormone, luteinising hormone, human chorionic gonadotropin, oestrogen, progesterone, relaxin, placental growth factor, human placental lactogen, oxytocin, cortisol, endorphins, and prolactin.

High levels of prolactin in the body prepare us for bonding and protection. The hormone acts to produce breastmilk and breast tissue for feeding. It is sometimes referred to as the 'mothering hormone' because it can increase the physiological desire to bond and protect your baby. Oxytocin, or the 'love hormone' as it is commonly known, is also responsible for the process of lactation as well as stimulating the uterus to contract during labour and birth. It is also responsible for how your brain develops a sense of trust, bonding, sexual arousal and recognition.

When you experience baby loss the levels of hormones do not magically return to your pre-pregnancy levels. Your body has been gearing up to protect and nurture a life, and significant changes occur in the brain to help you fulfil that role. As we know from menstruation, one of the biggest issues with hormones is their physical invisibility compared to their emotional impact. Baby loss impacts families and partners in many different ways, but the pregnant mother has to contend not only with the devastation of their loss and grief, but also with a whole body transformation as they learn to live with hormones that are geared up for a function that can no longer be fulfilled.

After your baby is born or your pregnancy ends your hormones will begin to return to their pre pregnancy level. This happens at different rates for different people and for each hormone. You may experience a very sudden drop in oestrogen and progesterone levels, which can contribute to low mood, anxiety and in some cases postnatal depression. These hormonal dips come alongside changes in your hormone levels caused by grief and your body's response to shock and trauma. Physically and mentally there is a lot going on and every day you may feel something entirely new.

What to do?

- Remember that your hormones will begin to regulate in the days and weeks after you have given birth or experienced pregnancy loss. They will not be like this forever.
- Be gentle and kind to yourself – permit yourself to feel whatever arises and don't try to 'think your way out' of what you are feeling.
- Use all the support that is available. If you feel more

comfortable staying in a hospital or birth centre and this is an option, allow yourself to be cared for over the first few days.

- Hormones can have a significant impact on your emotions, particularly in the days immediately after you give birth or experience loss. Your grief and potential shock will also give rise to additional hormones which will amplify your emotional response.
- Get a postnatal doula. Doula UK is a great starting point and they also have an access fund for people who cannot afford a doula. Getting some practical and emotional support from a trained doula might help you through the first few days.
- Eat healthy food. You may not feel like eating anything, and you may have sickness or a total aversion to food. Healthy food helps your body to get rid of the hormones that are not being used. Ask someone to make you something healthy and nourishing.
- Avoid numbing measures such as alcohol and drugs if possible. Your body needs to recover and as much as you may desperately want to ease your pain, these will not aid your hormonal recovery.
- Talk to your midwife about spending time with your baby if this is possible and what you want to do. If you experienced loss after a termination or early pregnancy, find support by talking to somebody on one of the helplines listed in the resource section of this book.
- You may wish to take some herbal remedies, prescribed pain killers or explore alternative therapies or treatments to help your body eliminate excess hormones.

Bleeding, cramping and vaginal health

After you give birth, at whatever stage of pregnancy, you will experience bleeding afterwards. This bleeding is called lochia and is more than just blood – it includes mucus and amniotic fluid. Speak in detail with your midwife about what level of blood loss is normal and ensure that you tell somebody immediately if your blood loss is substantial or has large clots, or if you feel faint or dizzy or generally unwell (beyond the emotional pain that you are feeling). Your bleeding will slow over the days or weeks, usually stopping completely within five to six weeks and sometimes lasting for as little as a week. You can wear maternity pads or regular pads to absorb the blood as the flow changes. Bleeding after loss can be a constant, stark reminder of what you have just experienced, and in addition to the emotional turmoil you will need to ensure that you keep yourself healthy and rested to recover. If you have had a vaginal delivery you may be experiencing some soreness, and you may have had stitches or tears and these need to be kept clean and soothed. You may experience afterpains as your uterus contracts, depending on what stage of pregnancy you were at. The sensation of cramping can be as mild as a period cramp or more severe and feel like birth contractions. It will take some time for your uterus to return to its normal size. This can be extremely challenging if you have reached later stages of pregnancy. You may continue to look pregnant for some weeks after your baby loss and this can lead to some people assuming that you are still pregnant. If you decide to go out to places where you may see people who will ask about your pregnancy, be prepared about how you will inform anybody who asks about what has happened. I have known couples choose to make their first public appearances away from their usual communities while the visible signs of pregnancy are still present. This is not to silence you: it is to protect you from having to relay your painful experience on your first venture outside. Of course, if you feel strong enough you can go wherever you want to – you are not responsible for protecting anybody else from the reality of what you have experienced.

What to do?

- Monitor your bleeding and talk to somebody if you experience anything that concerns you.
- Remember that you can ask for support and help with anything that you need.
- Keep in mind that your bleeding will slow over the next few days. Again, this is not something you are going to have to deal with for a long time. Be kind and patient with yourself.
- If you require assistance with bathroom activities, do not be afraid to ask. Sometimes the fear of being alone, even going to the toilet, might feel too much. Your doula, partner, friend or midwife will happily support you, and coming to the bathroom with you, even if just for company, is a perfectly reasonable request.
- Try pouring some warm water over your vulva and into the toilet as you urinate to alleviate any discomfort.
- Ask for pain relief if you need it. Your midwife or doctor will talk to you about what they recommend for your pain.

Lactation and breastmilk

In most cases lactation will start no earlier than 12 weeks' gestation, but of course there are exceptions to this. You may have previously fed, or still be feeding another child, and lactation may begin earlier in your pregnancy, or never have stopped. You may have experienced baby loss at full term or as neonatal loss and had the experience of a few days of feeding your baby. Some women, experiencing the heartbreak of the sudden death of their baby, will have had a substantial period of breastfeeding and may have a regular pattern of feeding their baby. After the loss of a multiple breastfeeding your other babies may trigger your grief as you imagine or yearn for the chance to feed your missing baby.

If you experience loss in the later stages of pregnancy you may experience engorgement of your breasts as your milk arrives in the days after birth. Your body is geared up to feed your baby and this can be both physically and emotionally challenging. You should get very clear advice and support from your midwife about lactation after loss. There are ways for your milk supply to be medically stopped, using a type of medication called dopamine agonists (unsuitable for some medical conditions), and there are ways to manage ceasing lactation without medication. For some women, especially those who've suffered the sudden death of their baby, ending lactation is another grieving process. Your loss may be amplified by the process of ceasing to lactate and there may be multiple experiences of grief as you reflect on both your baby and your feeding relationship.

One option is to continue with lactation and donate your breastmilk to other babies. This can be supported by your midwife or in liaison with your local milk bank. Contact details for these are in the further resources section of this book. Perhaps milk donation is a new concept for you – it is a valid and lifesaving choice to make, and it is right for some women and not for others. In milk donation you express your breastmilk and donate it to feed premature or poorly babies whose mothers are unable to feed them themselves. It is a profound gift to another baby, but it is always a choice and one that you can make and then back away from if you want to, once you know more about it. I encourage doulas and birth workers to research milk donation in order to present this as a choice for those you are supporting: the decision requires action relatively quickly, so if parents do not know that it is an option, it may be too late.

What to do?

- Ensure that you speak to your midwife about lactation and how you wish to proceed.
- If you are choosing to stop lactation you can receive guidance on how to express small amounts to bring relief to your breasts, while ensuring that you do not continue to stimulate your supply.
- When breasts feel tender or sore you can bring relief through medication from your midwife or doctor, by placing cold green cabbage leaves onto engorged breasts and by taking a warm shower to release a small amount of milk.
- Ensure that you consider donation carefully and remember that if donation feels right in the first instance you can always change your mind later.
- There are services listed in this book for preserving small amounts of your breastmilk in keepsakes. Some women have found comfort in creating items such as jewellery with a drop or two of their milk.
- If you experience pain in your breasts, or symptoms of fever, speak to your midwife or health visitor or contact one of the services providing lactation advice after loss listed in the resource section.
- Reverse pressure softening is a technique that can help with engorgement and avoiding mastitis (an

inflammation of breast tissue that sometimes involves an infection) and help milk flow if it needs to.

Carefully alleviating engorgement can aid the slowing of milk supply.

Placenta

Depending on how you came to baby or pregnancy loss you may have been able to birth your baby's placenta. The placenta has varying significance for parents, with some attaching great significance to its role in helping to grow and nurture their baby, while others do not see it in the same terms. The placenta is an organ that develops in your uterus during pregnancy. It provides oxygen and nutrients to your growing baby and removes waste products from your baby's blood. The placenta attaches to the wall of your uterus, and your baby's umbilical cord arises from it.

After the birth of a live baby many parents choose to delay the clamping of the cord between baby and placenta, allowing for all of the blood in the cord to be transferred to their baby. I have known clients who have birthed stillborn babies who have asked that the placenta not be detached from the baby at all, so it is kept with them as they are buried or cremated. In many circumstances of baby loss you may not have this option, but if it is important to you, talk to your midwife about your wishes for the placenta.

Some women face complications with their placenta that mean that after the birth of their baby they must go to theatre to have all or part of the placenta removed. This experience can be an additional challenge and trauma for a woman who has already experienced baby loss. Having to face a theatre procedure while in shock and grieving loss may amplify your physical or emotional grief. Remembering that your placenta story is also a part of your birth story may allow you to share and explore your birth more fully when reviewing the events around your loss.

What to do?

- Remember that your placenta is an important part of your birth and loss experience.
- If you have preferences for what happens to or with your placenta, you have every right to discuss these options with your doula, midwife or bereavement midwife.
- If you have to go to theatre for a manual removal of the placenta, ask your doula or partner to ask to attend with you so that you have emotional support during the procedure. It may not be within the guidelines of all trusts for this to be possible, but having attended with several of my own clients I know that it is an option.
- Your placenta has played an important role in the development of your baby. If you have a relationship of significance with the placenta and wish to explore options for what happens to it after you leave the hospital you have every right to ask these questions and consider what is best for you.

Your body after loss

Our bodies change significantly during pregnancy and can also alter as we attempt conception. Depending on whether you knew of your pregnancy and at what time in your journey your loss occurred you may have noticed a few changes or very significant ones. After your loss you will continue to experience changes as your uterus returns to its pre-pregnant size and your body learns to adapt to not having the baby (or babies) that it anticipated. Being gentle with yourself and your body during this time is important to ensure that you recover physically and mentally. You may not feel able to eat or drink as usual, but keeping your physical strength is important. In the weeks and months after your birth you might want to undertake postnatal exercise. Often women undertake postnatal exercise in groups with other new mothers and after an experience of baby loss these may feel excluding or impossible to face. I am sorry that there are not more available classes that are inclusive of baby loss, and I encourage anybody working in postnatal exercise to increase their understanding of how to hold space for mothers who have experienced loss. But for those of you wishing that you could find the techniques to recover without having to face a room of new mums, know that you can contact postnatal instructors for private sessions, or use online resources to understand what is happening to your body postnatally and what is best for you as it recovers.

For some women, baby loss may result in the additional loss of a healthy relationship with their own body. Negative words such as failure, barren, useless or broken have been shared with me by women who have come to view their body extremely negatively or in a negative way. Your body is incredible, truly magnificent, and worthy of adoration and love. Simply reading these words will not be enough to heal you of any negative associations that you have made with your body in relation to your loss, but I encourage you to reach out for support, perhaps to a therapist or bereavement specialist, to acknowledge these feelings to help you recover a sense of belief in your body.

What to do?

- Notice if you have negative associations with your body and/or its ability.
- Speak to somebody about what you are feeling about your body.
- Consider having a 'closing the bones' ceremony to nurture your body and begin to heal from your birth.
- Ask somebody to prepare nutritious food and drink for you and ensure that you stay hydrated and fed in the days and weeks after your loss.
- Consider postnatal exercise once you have recovered physically and have stopped bleeding. Speak to local instructors about what they offer and how they can work with you.

Contraception and future pregnancy

Depending on your loss you will be given guidance about the right time to consider future conception. You do not have to go on to have future pregnancies, and if you do, you will not be 'replacing' your baby. However, it is important to consider contraception if you intend to have sex. Becoming pregnant again may carry risks for you based on your loss experience, and you need to understand these risks and how they can be mitigated. Being emotionally prepared for future pregnancies is also important, and timing future conception to allow for your grief to be realised is important. It can be extremely healing to have a baby after loss. Considering this immediately after loss may feel absurd, but if you are having sex and do not want to become pregnant again while you grieve your loss contraception and planning are important. An unexpected pregnancy shortly after an experience of loss can bring fear and trauma that adds to the weight of your grief, so ensure you talk about and consider what a pregnancy would be like and make informed choices about what is right for you and your partner.

The fourth trimester is usually emotionally and physically challenging for all women, so for you to endure the changes in your body without your baby can feel impossible and lonely. Your body is longing to do something that it cannot physically do and waiting to heal can be tough. I am sorry our society does not support you better; you deserve as much support as any other new mother. My hope is that with the help of charities, support services, peer support and information you will find a way to navigate the fourth trimester with support.

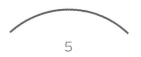

5

Offering support
after loss

There is no pill that can replace human connection, no pharmacy that can fill the prescription for compassionate others. The answer to human suffering lies both between us and within us.

Dr. Joanne Cacciatore author of *Bearing the Unbearable:*
Love, loss, and the heartbreaking path of grief

When somebody that you know or are in a relationship with experiences baby loss or the loss of a pregnancy it can be extremely difficult to know what to do and say. Hopefully, this book will suggest ways that you can build empathic compassion into your support for their grief. Of course, your own grief also matters and if you are the other parent, or a close family relation, you may also feel the heartbreak of loss. You also had hopes, dreams, ideas and love for the baby, and you will be carrying your loss and grief alongside a deep desire to help. There are some ways in which we can better support people just by thinking about our language, what we do, how we work towards including people and continuing to show up for those who need us.

Language of support

> *Lots of people say things like 'at least you have a child already, focus on her'. Lots of people ask how many children I have, and I want to say two, even though I haven't, not anymore, but I did. I've birthed two babies.*
> Alison, mother to B2

Words give feelings, experiences and events credibility. They are also limiting and when we are dealing with grief, they are complicated. Both the words that you need to feel understood and the words that people choose to use when supporting your grief can be clumsy and inaccurate. Grief is, as we have seen, a matter of the heart and not the head and trying to find the right words is extremely challenging.

Many people do not know what to say to a person who has experienced baby or pregnancy loss. It is probably worth stating that there are no right words. There is no fix to death and loss, and while recovery and healing may come, it will not be because of somebody saying the right words. However, there is value in exploring our language around grief, and there are particular approaches that may go a long way to ensuring that we foster healing rather than causing further hurt.

Non-violent communication is predicated on approaching communication with an intention to 'connect not correct' and this is a useful reminder for us all when finding the words to support somebody in grief. Saying anything that begins with 'at least…' does not connect to the grief, it aims to correct it with a solution. 'At least you know you can get pregnant' does not heal grief for a pregnancy loss, and 'At least you have your other two children' does not connect to the loss of a much-wanted baby. There is no place for 'at least' in baby loss. Similarly, the idea that 'Everything happens for a reason' does nothing to acknowledge the sadness and tragedy of baby loss. When you are supporting a person in their grief, try to ask yourself if you are trying to connect with or correct/fix/reassure them. Unfortunately, there is no reassurance or hope in the immediacy of baby loss, nothing can return that baby to the arms of their parents. Meeting your friend or partner with words that allow and acknowledge their grief presents the opportunity for connection. Try mirroring their language and emotions with your words: 'It is so sad, I can see your pain and I am here to hold it with you'. If they refer to their baby by name, ask if you can use the name too.

Speculation about where a baby has gone should also be led by the person who has experienced the loss first-hand. Do not project your own perspective of the baby 'being in a better place', or 'being in heaven'. There is no better place for a newborn baby than within the loving arms of its parents, and no reassurance is given by presenting a 'better' option. While the intention may be to offer hope and positivity, unless these suggestions are offered by the parent then they are not welcome.

I got back to work and a colleague came up and put his hand on my shoulder, 'At least you made it further along in this pregnancy, you'll get there next time' and he patted me sympathetically and walked on. That was me done in for the day, honestly, I had just lost my baby and he couldn't even just say the word sorry. Life has to move on, next baby, next baby… sorry but I am not as mechanical as that. I wanted that baby, not the next one.
Jono, father to Fig

Whenever you are supporting somebody with loss or grief, reminding yourself to check your intention, language and behaviour against the following list can be really useful.

The best ways

- Be supportive, try not to fix the grief
- Speak about feelings
- Be non-active, do not tell people what they should do
- Do not try to change a person's feelings
- Recognise the loss
- Do not time-limit grief
- Seek connection, not correction
- Mirror language used by the person experiencing grief

The worst ways

- Trying to fix or move on from the loss
- Being directive in nature and offering solutions
- Attempting to explain or justify loss
- Being judgemental
- Putting a timeline on loss
- Being corrective rather than connective
- Comparing or lessening the loss

Actions of support

My doula mentor recently used the beautiful phrase '*just to be in companionable silence with you would be enough*' when communicating her wish to be with her friends. That 'companionable silence' is so often enough. To be with and alongside others, not speaking or trying to create conversation or find the right words. If you are supporting a person who is experiencing grief after baby or pregnancy loss, perhaps just being there, being present, is enough. Nothing you can do will fix the pain that they are in and you showing up and being with them may well be exactly what they need.

After baby loss it may be that parents want to be alone for some time, or they may be desperate for company. Approaching what is right can be challenging as the grieving parents may not know exactly what they want. Saying 'you know where I am' can be tricky, because this does not provide a specific opportunity for the griever to accept or decline your support. Being very clear about your offer of support allows people to give a clear yes or no. You could send a message saying 'Would you like company this afternoon, I am free from 1pm and can come to you. Fine to say yes or no.' This allows a clear response and gives them permission to decline. Continuing to provide these clear offers of time and support requires little from the person at the centre of the ring of grief.

Offering food that can be stored, frozen or kept may be gratefully received. You do not need to impose, but you can drop food round with a card or leave it in a cool box on the doorstep. Cards in the post can also be very meaningful.

We opened the door to a huge box of food and comforting items and we both just felt so loved. Our friends had given us everything we needed for those first days and they had done it without interrupting our privacy. Anna Dale

Ask your friend if they would like to tell you about their baby or birth experience, and if they have photographs that they would like to show you. These stories and details may be hard to hear, but can go a long way to acknowledging that you see that your friend has just given birth and may wish to share this with somebody. If the baby has a name, use it, create keepsakes with it on, address cards to them and write words for them. In the acknowledgment of their existence we can support grief to be held with compassion.

Money can be a worry for some grieving parents, and although they may continue to be eligible for some maternity pay and/or benefits they may be concerned about the months ahead. If it is within your means to offer financial support to your friend in some way, consider how to best approach this and make an offer. Pay for them to take a holiday when they feel ready, or give them the money they need for fuel or food over the next few weeks. If you cannot afford to allocate money, you could quietly ask a few friends to donate and offer the money towards something of the parents' choosing. You could ask if there is a charity that the parents would like you to donate to, or raise funds for, as a legacy to their loss.

Partners and close relatives could offer to undertake the process of unsubscribing the mother from pregnancy forums or groups on social media. Obviously, this should be done with permission, but it is a very thoughtful action that can alleviate some of the pain associated with returning to social interactions which may be full of pregnancy related updates.

Ensuring that the person at the centre of grief is being supported with telling people is important. There will be certain people that they want to speak to and others that they don't. Ask first and then offer to tell local people who they may come into contact with. This might be the owners of local cafés or classes, clubs or social groups. Always ask first and remember to deliver the news with sensitivity and care, and look after yourself by seeking support from others, as repeating sad news can take its toll.

The single most important action is to keep remembering. There is nothing more significant than continuing to hold space for grief long after the event of loss. Remember anniversaries and mark them, and continue to offer to be there for your friend as they navigate the next weeks, months and years of their life. Just as you would a mother or father of a living child, remember to continue to check how they are feeling, healing, and coping.

Support for siblings

If you have experienced baby or pregnancy loss and you also have other children or stepchildren, cousins or close friends who are young, it is important that they are supported to grieve in a way that is appropriate to their age and understanding. However you refer to the loss of your baby, it is important that younger people are able to understand the concept of death in a way that provides them with a safe environment in which to explore their feelings towards it. Some of the language used to describe baby loss, such as 'sleeping' or 'angel' or 'up in heaven' may not be appropriate for your other child. If they are young they may misinterpret well-meaning language and not fully understand that their sibling is not coming back. Exploring the concept of death with a young child can be confusing, and it can be challenging to find the words to support a child without offering them hope. We have to simultaneously ensure that they feel safe, while allowing them to understand the enormous concept of the end of life. Try to acknowledge your child's grief and allow it. Let them be sad and cry, or be angry, and where possible include them in rituals to remember their sibling. Try to encourage them to keep the memory alive within the family.

At the same time as wanting to keep the memory of your loss alive, there is a need to ensure that you don't cultivate an image of your child's sibling as forever perfect. You will have days when your living children are being annoying, or having mood swings, tantrums, needs and moments of selfishness. It is important that as your child grows older, they understand that they are not being compared to their lost sibling. Sometimes a living sibling may feel resentful of their lost sibling as they see how their memory is protected by a veil of perfection while they are being told off or challenged about their behaviour. Talk honestly and openly with your other children. Let them know that their sibling would have had difficult days too, and remind them that you are so grateful to have them in your life.

Raising other children while experiencing grief can be emotionally and physically exhausting, so allow other people to support you. This is a practical way in which you can involve your friends and family. Ask them to take younger children on days out – it will be easier for them to create an environment of fun and enjoyment without being so immediately impacted by grief. Older children and teenagers might benefit from having a relative that specifically directs their support towards them. Ask an aunty or friend to regularly check in with your older child, allowing them to talk openly about their grief away from your feelings.

Being sad in the company of your other children is okay. Seeing your grief will permit them their own and you are showing your child that it is alright to be sad and upset. Neither parent needs to hide their grief from other siblings. Children are extremely sensitive to emotional changes and if you suppress your grief, they may blame themselves for the underlying, unspoken sadness in your home. If they know that your sadness relates to your loss, not to them, it will allow them to explore their grief without feeling responsible.

On the way home, I was clutching my baby scan picture, looking at this perfect shape and knowing he/she wasn't alive anymore. Once home I was greeted by my two-year-old and immediately I just collapsed on the floor with utter grief. She went and got me a daisy flower from the garden to cheer me up!

Every year I light two candles on a special tree that I've planted in my garden, and although my husband doesn't it's something that I do. I never got to meet those babies, but I have my scan pictures in a special box with the daisy flower that my daughter picked from the garden. It never leaves you the sense of loss, it will always be a reminder of what could have been I suppose. Joanne Sieber

Rainbow babies

You may have heard people refer to a baby born after a previous loss as a rainbow baby. The symbolism of the rainbow bringing hope after the storm brings comfort to many parents when and if they decide to have future babies. The availability of a word that has become widely known and accepted offers a context for people to understand that this new baby comes after a time of great loss and grief. As with all words, referring to your future baby as a rainbow baby may not feel right for you.

However, you may find your new pregnancy referred to as a rainbow baby at antenatal appointments with your midwife. In recent years butterfly, rainbow or teardrop stickers have been added to pregnancy notes to signify to midwives that you are pregnant after a loss. The aim is that your care is then more personalised to take into account what has happened to you in the past.

Having a baby after a previous loss or losses can bring emotions of guilt, increased sadness for your previous loss, or resentment towards a new baby who survived when your other baby did not. These feelings can be really confusing and isolating, and it is important that you feel able to vocalise them with your partner, midwife, counsellor or peer support network. They are part of your grief, which is your response to loss, and all the feelings should be welcomed and worked with rather than ignored or suppressed. Remember that you are not in control of your grief, you are learning to live with it and where feelings arise, they require acknowledgement and compassion to adapt into your life going forward.

Support for fathers and other partners

Grief after baby or pregnancy loss will impact everybody who was expecting the new life, the healthy child, or the delivery of all multiples. Baby loss impacts men and women, partners and other close relatives, and everybody's grief is valid. I have tried to make this book relevant for all people, regardless of your immediacy of relationship to the loss, but if you are intimately connected to the person giving birth, or you are the other biological parent of the baby, your grief may have additional dimensions. You will be experiencing loss in a different way to your partner or co-parent. If you did not carry the baby or pregnancy in your body, or if you weren't the person undergoing fertility treatment, you may feel that your loss comes 'second'. Certainly with early pregnancy loss it can be challenging to conceptualise the degree of loss – you may not have had chance to accept, bond with or imagine the life growing within your partner, and you may not have begun to consider yourself as a parent. Indeed, in the case of a miscarriage prior to knowledge of the pregnancy you may come to learn about loss before you learn about life.

Supporting an intimate partner who has experienced physical changes within their body requires care and compassion, patience and support. If you have found yourself in the position of caring for another person's physical needs after baby or pregnancy loss you may not have taken the time to look after yourself. As the second parent the ring of grief can be a vital tool. Ask a close friend to be there just for you, perhaps by providing telephone support or daily check-ins. They can be there for you so you can 'dump out' emotionally.

I lost my son when he was six days old and that was five years ago. I have another son now, but I remember my firstborn every day. It is kind of hard as a Dad because people haven't seen me pregnant, people don't expect me to weep at my desk and run out of meetings, so I have had to pretend and do a lot of 'holding it together'. Those that do know just don't have any words, so they say nothing. I have had to be there for my wife and to be honest my feelings have just been my own a lot of the time. We remember him together, but I just had to be strong, and really, I was and sometimes still am, broken. David, father to Sim

If you have to return to work after baby loss and leave your partner at home, this will likely feel strange and potentially painful. It may also mean that you return to 'normal' life sooner than your partner, and begin to find distractions that divert your mental energy away from dwelling in a space of grief and loss. Parents having to return to work very soon after loss may feel that they have little or no time to unpick and work with their grief. Asking your colleagues to be supportive may feel hard, but it is important that you create an environment of understanding within your workplace. It may be that your colleagues do not know how to support you, and perhaps asking for some flexibility in your working hours or location for a few months is appropriate. Your work may not allow such alterations, and while asking for support is encouraged, many workplaces are not accommodating of emotional struggles. Building into your daily routine an option to pause, perhaps at the end of the day before you step over the threshold of home, to check in with and reflect on how your grief is manifesting is worthwhile. Perhaps you could find a spot to stop each day for 15 minutes prior to coming home and resuming your supportive role.

Dads can feel ignored or shunned from the grief experience, particularly in the hospital environment, which can feel entirely orientated towards the care of the woman or birthing person. There are many improvements that can be made to better support Dads and other partners. SANDS provides excellent support and peer groups for partners and fathers, and while going to certain groups as a couple is an excellent option, consider finding a support group just for you and your grief. SANDS also has a booklet called 'Mainly for Fathers' which provides valuable insight and information on your grief, rights, work return and support groups.

Being honest with yourself and your partner will be so beneficial. Talk about what is going on for you and ensure that you are working not only to support your partner, but also to allow your own grief. You have also lost your child and you are absolutely entitled to your grief and sadness.

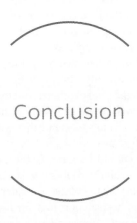

Conclusion

Baby loss and pregnancy loss can lead to some of the deepest pain, some of the saddest, most torturous narratives of our lives. It is often quiet, often lonely and it cannot be 'fixed'. Grief is never wrong, nor is it ever better or worse than somebody else's – it is an unquantifiable response which manifests differently for us all. What I have come to understand is that every single experience of loss needs to be supported at the pace of the people at the centre of the ring of grief. Your feelings are your feelings because they are your feelings and that is enough. If we can meet every person in a place of deep empathy, setting aside our own opinions, setting aside our own judgement, our expectations and fears, if we can see and be with the pain that is there, maybe this will go some way towards our culture speaking openly and safely about baby loss. Maybe, if we can recognise that we have grown into a society that isn't giving death the same weight as life, a society that avoids talking about death because we have lost the language for it, then we can move forward to find more compassion and courage. It is okay that we don't know how to do that yet, but as a birth worker and woman who has experienced the loss of her own baby, I know that I commit to a path of always learning, always seeing a way that I can be more present with the grief of others. And to those of you who are experiencing loss, recent or historic, I hope that you will heal, in your own unique way, and that within that healing one day you will find peace.

What stands out most to me is the benefit of finding support, and particularly peer support. For those of you working to support birth, please consider it your duty to understand how to best support loss, for it is never far away. Researching and contacting local support groups is a vital part of our responsibility as birth workers. I have provided details of support that is available nationally in England, and there will be more locally. Signposting friends and family, clients and partners to the support that they need is important, and ensuring that you receive support when you are experiencing grief is also necessary. I applaud the work of all these organisations: they are often run on a shoestring and are standing alongside thousands of women and birthing people and their families every year.

Your hopes, expectations, dreams and wishes for the life that has been lost are your reminder of the love that you can give and share. That you have pain alongside this love is heartbreaking and grief can be relentless, returning again and again in new and different ways. I believe that you can find the support and the care to navigate your grief and move towards healing and recovery, and that you can do this while also keeping the memory of your baby alive in your heart. I am so sorry for your loss, and so grateful that you have found the strength to engage in how you might continue with the life ahead of you.

> *Every time I witness a strong person, I want to know: What dark did you conquer in your story? Mountains do not rise without earthquakes.* Katherine MacKenett

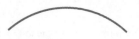

Acknowledgements

Writing this book has allowed me to have 190 of the hardest and most humbling exchanges of my life. To every person who shared their experience of love and loss and their babies with me, I'm so grateful. My heartfelt gratitude to my All4Maternity tribe. To my maternity heroes and mentors Maddie, Milli, Sheena and Brigid, you've transformed my capacity. To Elsie and Naava, Nikki and Ellie and Mum for your insight. To Clare and Dave, and Luna for inspiring the purpose. To Tess for holding and evolving my soul in therapy. Thank you Sam, Suki and Oslo for letting me write, cry and write more, through a challenging lockdown. My love and thanks to Will, Rosie, Weibka and Sam for always being my people. To Susan and Martin for the faith and encouragement and for making this book come into being.

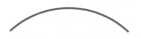

Further reading and resources

Books

Personal accounts of baby loss

Ask me his Name by Elle Wright
Saying Goodbye by Zoe Clark-Coates
Life after Baby Loss by Nicola Gaskin
Mothers in Waiting by Crystal Bowman and Meghan Bowman

Books for children about loss and grief

The Paper Dolls by Julia Donaldson
This Book is for all Kids but especially my sister Libby: Libby Died by James Simon
The Invisible String by Patrice Karst

Grief

On Grief and Grieving by Elisabeth Kubler-Ross and David Kessler
On Death and Dying by Elisabeth Kubler-Ross

Bearing the Unbearable: Love, Loss and the heart-breaking path of grief by Joanne Cacciatore

Understanding Your Grief by Alan D. Wolfelt

Yoga for Grief and Loss by Karla Helbert

The Grief Recovery Handbook by John W. James and Russell Friedman

Life after loss

Bereaved parents and their continued bonds – love after loss by Catherine Seigal

It's okay that you're not okay by Megan Divine

Life After Birth by Diane Speier. This book is for parents with living babies. It has good content on life with loss but may be triggering.

Trauma and recovery

Trauma and human existence by Robert D. Stolorow

The Body Keeps the Score: Brain Mind and Body in healing trauma by Bessel Van der Kolk

True Refuge by Tara Brach

Trauma, PTSD, Grief and Loss by Michael Dubi

Ritual and ceremony

Benedictus by John O'Donohoe

Good Grief Rituals: Tools for Healing by Elaine Childs-Gowell

Specific birth and pregnancy issues

Polyamory and Pregnancy by Jessica Burde

Reproductive Justice by Loretta J. Ross and Rickie Solinger

Baby loss helplines

Picking up the phone to speak to somebody can feel scary. Please remember that helpline support is offered by peer supporters. Nobody will expect you to share anything if you are unwilling, and if you are in desperate need, isolated or feeling overwhelmed taking the step to get peer support can be extremely helpful.

If you have experienced *pregnancy loss* in any circumstance call:

Miscarriage Association – pregnancy loss helpline
   01924 200799

If you have experienced *pregnancy loss, stillbirth, or any circumstance of baby loss* call:

Tommy's helpline
   0800 0147 800 www.tommys.org

SANDS national helpline
   0808 164 3331 www.sands.org.uk

If you have experienced the *sudden or unexpected death of a baby or young child* call:

Lullaby Trust helpline 0808 802 6868
   www.lullabytrust.org.uk

Additional online and telephone services and support:

At A Loss Online loss and bereavement signposting
   www.ataloss.org

Nova Foundation Resources and Support for Baby Loss
   www.novafoundation.org.uk/findingbabylosssupport

A Child of Mine – Help for Bereaved Parents Practical information and guidance after the death of a child.
Helpline 07803 751229
hello@achildofmine.org.uk | www.achildofmine.org.uk

Antenatal Results and Choices (ARC) Information and support to parents before, during and after antenatal screening.
Helpline: 0845 077 2290 or 0207 713 7486
info@arc-uk.org | www.arc-uk.org

Bliss for babies born premature or sick
020 7378 1122 | ask@bliss.org.uk | www.bliss.org.uk

Care for the Family Provides parent support, family support and bereavement support. Has a Christian ethos.
029 2081 0800 | mail@cff.org.uk | www.careforthefamily.org.uk

Child Bereavement UK – CBUK Supports families and educates professionals when a child of any age has died or is dying and when a child is bereaved. Offers free face-to-face bereavement support in Buckinghamshire, Cheshire, Cumbria, Glasgow, Leeds, Milton Keynes, east London, west London.
National helpline: 0800 02 888 40
support@childbereavementuk.org
Live chat via www.childbereavementuk.org

The Child Death Helpline Helpline that offers support to anyone affected by the death of a child of any age, under any circumstances, however recent or long ago. Free interpretation for languages other than English.
Freephone 0800 282 986 or 0808 800 6019
contact@childdeathhelpline.org | childdeathhelpline.org.uk

The Compassionate Friends Bereaved parents and their families offering understanding, support, and encouragement to others after the death of a child or children.
National helpline: 0345 123 2304
Northern Ireland helpline: 0288 77 88 016
helpline@tcf.org.uk www.tcf.org.uk

Cruse Bereavement Care Support for people bereaved, in any way, whatever their age, nationality or belief. Cruse has a dedicated website for young people: www.hopeagain.org.uk
Helpline: 0808 808 1677
helpline@cruse.org.uk | www.cruse.org.uk

UK Association of Milk Banking Milk banks in the UK strive to look after donors and make the process of donating milk as simple as possible.
www.ukamb.org/donate-milk

Saying Goodbye Provides Cathedral remembrance services for anyone whose baby has died at any stage of pregnancy, at birth or in infancy.
0845 293 8027 | info@sayinggoodbye.org
www.sayinggoodbye.org | www.mariposatrust.org

TAMBA Bereavement Support Group (part of the Twins and Multiple Births Association) Support for parents who have lost a twin/multiple or both twins/all multiples.
Helpline: 01252 332 344 | support-team@tamba.org.uk
www.tamba.org.uk/bereavement

Pregnancy After Loss Support (PALS) This organisation is based in the US, but they offer a lot of online resources and support for people who are pregnant after a previous loss. www.pregnancyafterlosssupport.org

British Association for Counselling and Psychotherapy (BACP)
How to find a private therapist. Fees will apply for
services.
01455 883300 | bacp@bacp.co.uk | www.bacp.co.uk

*British Association for Behavioural and Cognitive Therapies
(CBT)* Details of all officially accredited CBT therapists.
www.babcp.com

UK Council for Psychotherapy (UKCP) The UK's leading
professional body for the education, training and
accreditation of psychotherapists and psychotherapeutic
counsellors. Most will charge a fee.
020 7014 9955 | info@ukcp.org.uk
www.psychotherapy.org.uk

Grief Chat Telephone and online grief chat support.
www.griefchat.co.uk

Doula UK Find a Doula service with details of all birth and
postnatal doulas, their areas of expertise and contact
information, detailed by area. Fees are charged for
services, access fund available.
www.doula.org.uk

IMUK Independent Midwives in the UK. Find a midwife
who can offer you advice and guidance tailored to your
individual needs. Fees are charged for services.
www.imuk.org.uk

Birthrights Provides advice and information to women and
campaign for respectful and safe maternity care that
protects women's fundamental rights.
www.birthrights.org.uk

3-Step Rewind The 3-step Rewind involves working with you to lift the heavy feelings and symptoms that can remain after a difficult or traumatic birth, postnatal or breastfeeding experience, or any other perinatal trauma. www.elliethedoula.com/trauma-recovery

Closing the Bones Closing the Bones is a ritual, massage and ceremony offered to support a woman's recovery after birth. www.closingthebonesmassage.com

Birth and loss doula Author Kay King's website for booking or speaking about her doula services for parents wishing to access a loss-informed doula service. www.birthandloss.uk

Supporting Every Birth An interactive workshop created for doulas and birth workers looking at supporting both clients and themselves through all birth journeys including baby loss. nurturingbirth.co.uk/retreats-and-workshops/supporting-every-birth

Grief Recovery Method Learn how to move beyond death and other losses. Find a specialist. www.griefrecoverymethod.co.uk | 01234 862218

Non-Violent Communication NVC is the language of connection; a totally learnable, practical way to bring empathy, honesty, strength, and compassion into our personal and professional relationships. www.nvc-uk.com

Women's Aid National support and resources for women and children experiencing domestic abuse. www.womensaid.org.uk

Refuge National Domestic Abuse Helpline – 0808 2000 247

Podcasts

Listening to a regular podcast on topics relating to baby loss, healing practices and techniques or social action can be useful after your loss. You can search for these podcasts on all main platforms and choose an episode.

Tara Brach Tara Brach's teachings blend Western psychology and Eastern spiritual practices, mindful attention to our inner life, and a full, compassionate engagement with our world.

The Fertility Podcast To educate and empower you about your fertility.

The Birth Activists Pregnancy, birth and baby topics with birth activists Samantha Gadsden, Becki Scott and guests.

Heal your Heart after Baby Loss The podcast for you if you want to heal, rebuild your life and make peace with losing a baby.

Sisters in Loss Podcast Miscarriage, pregnancy loss and infertility stories. Spotlights faith-filled black women who share their grief and loss stories and testimonies.

Social action after baby loss

When your life has been altered by an experience of pregnancy or baby loss, you may feel inspired or motivated to join in with social action, research and awareness-raising to help alleviate the future suffering of others. It is not your personal responsibility to change maternity standards or care or to campaign for increased awareness around baby loss, but if you feel that this is an area of interest, or you would like the legacy of your loss to be marked by a donation or campaign, consider getting in touch.

Five X More There is a five-fold difference in maternal mortality rates among women from black ethnic backgrounds and an almost two-fold difference among women from Asian ethnic backgrounds compared to white women. Five X More is a campaign set up to challenge and change this inequality.
www.fivexmore.com

White Ribbon Alliance UK When women are healthy so are their children, families, communities and countries. WRA understands the synergy between sexual, reproductive, maternal, newborn, child and adolescent health policies and services and implements holistic solutions.
www.whiteribbonalliance.org.uk

Baby Loss Awareness Baby Loss Awareness week happens every year in October in the UK. The website details lots of different ways in which you can get involved, support and aid the efforts of collective awareness raising.
www.babyloss-awareness.org

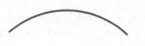

Index

Series editor: Susan Last

pinterandmartin.com